Menopause Doesn't Have to Suck

Science-Backed Solutions to Debunk Common Myths, Beat the Symptoms, Manage Perimenopause (and Beyond) with Humor!

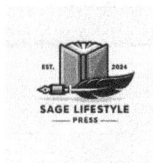

Sage Lifestyle Press

Menopause Doesn't Have to Suck

Disclaimer:
This book is intended for informational purposes only. The author is not a medical professional, and the information provided in this book should not be considered a substitute for professional medical advice, diagnosis, or treatment. Always seek the advice of your physician or other qualified health providers with any questions you may have regarding a medical condition. Never disregard professional medical advice or delay in seeking it because of something you have read in this book.

The author and publisher disclaim any liability or responsibility for any adverse effects or consequences resulting from the use of any suggestions, preparations, or procedures discussed in this book.

Printed in the United States of America

This 2026 edition has been updated with the latest research and insights on menopause, hormone therapy, and women's health.

Contents

Introduction

S o there I was, in the middle of a hot flash, feeling like I was auditioning for a low-budget action film called *Menopause: The Heat Is On.* If you're smiling, you've probably had one yourself or stood beside someone fanning her way through it. Menopause is an unpredictable ride filled with sudden drops, steep climbs, and a few scream-worthy turns. But here's the thing, it doesn't have to suck.

Menopause isn't just a biological event; it's a rite of passage. A stage that brings the potential for change, strength, and humor if you let it. The word itself might spark visions of sleepless nights, stubborn chin hairs, and a body that feels like it's running its own experiments. Behind those moments are truths worth uncovering and myths ready to fall away. This is a transformation, not a decline.

Many women lie awake wondering, *Am I losing my mind?* or, *will I ever fit into those jeans again?* You're far from alone. One in a hundred women reaches menopause before forty, and one in a thousand before thirty. Ten percent take time off work to manage symptoms, while a quarter experience them severely. These numbers aren't meant to alarm you. They remind you that you're part of a much larger sisterhood going through the same transition.

If you've ever whispered to a friend about brain fog or laughed until you cried over a hot flash in public, you already know how powerful shared stories can be. That sense of connection and those small moments of humor and honesty can turn an isolating experience into one of camaraderie. The goal is not to "get through it" quietly, but to understand what's happening and take charge of your well-being with knowledge and compassion.

Take Christine, for example. She's leading a presentation when heat rises from nowhere, turning her silk blouse into a battlefield. Certain she's imploding, she bolts to the restroom. There, she meets Sarah, a seasoned midlife warrior who offers advice and empathy. A few laughs later, Christine walks back out, armed with a mini fan and a little more perspective. One conversation, one moment of understanding, and everything feels a bit lighter.

Menopause can feel uncomfortable, confusing, but also surprisingly funny once you stop fighting it. With knowledge and support from other women, it becomes less about surviving and more about discovering what's next. You start to notice what your body needs: more rest, more movement, better boundaries, and a healthy dose of self-kindness.

This book combines science, humor, and lived experience to help you laugh, learn, and take charge. Inside, you'll find stories that sound like your own and practical tools that make symptoms easier to manage. The goal isn't perfection. It's confidence. And laughter helps. It lightens the load, rebuilds connection, and reminds you that you're still you.

You'll learn how hormones affect everything from sleep to mood and what actually works to feel like yourself again. Along the way, we'll look at modern resources such as apps, online groups, and tools that make this stage more manageable. We'll also talk about how to include the men in our lives who care about us and want to help. They're part of this story too.

If Christine found calm through humor and connection, you can too. Together, we'll replace embarrassment with understanding and isolation with community. You'll discover how self-advocacy, curiosity, and a willingness to laugh can make all the difference.

Welcome to a new chapter of life that's messy, real, and full of second chances. It's time to laugh through the hot flashes, listen to your body, and walk forward with confidence, grace, and maybe an extra shirt in your bag.

Your Exclusive Free Companion Resources

T hank you for getting your copy of ***Menopause Doesn't Have to Suck!***
I've created some special resources to help you feel informed, confident, and empowered through every stage of menopause.

Access your free downloads here:

Scan the QR code below:

Chapter One

The Real Deal: Menopause Without the Filter

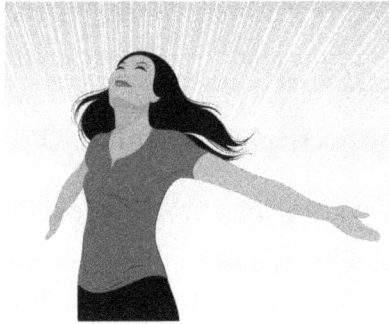

Menopause—it's a word that can trigger an eye-roll or a sigh of resignation in many women. Whether you're just beginning this adventure or have been trekking through it for some time, understanding menopause is like trying to read a mystery novel where the ending keeps changing. It's not just a chapter in your life; it's a book filled with plot twists, keeping you on your toes and ready for the unexpected.

Menopause comes with its own comedy and drama set, often flashing unexpectedly on your life's screen. Here's a scenario: You're addressing your colleagues in a work meeting, all composed and steady, when suddenly, you can't find your glasses. All eyes are on you as you shuffle papers and dig through your bag while all eyes are on you. You hear a subtle cough, look up, and see your boss motioning to the top of his head. You reach up, then feel your face fill with intense heat as you find your glasses softly perched within your flowing locks.

In this chapter, I'm here to debunk myths, sprinkle in some humor, and offer a reality check about this phase that's as inevitable as taxes. You'll discover what menopause means beyond the clichés and jokes and how it's not just a countdown to a distant land of gray hair and knitting needles.

Understanding Menopause: Myths vs. Realities

"Life doesn't end with menopause; it's the beginning of a new adventure. Strap in and enjoy the ride!" — ***Dame Helen Mirren***

Myth #1: Menopause Hits When You're Old

Hearing the word "menopause" might evoke images of grandmas and knitting circles, but that's the first misconception to debunk. Many women think of menopause as an event reserved for those in their twilight years. Surprise! It can start earlier than you think. Perimenopause, the transition to menopause, can start in your 30s or 40s, leading to a year without periods (Miller, 2024).

Imagine being in your prime, juggling career and family, and suddenly realizing that subtle changes are heralding this natural transition. It's not about your age; it's about your readiness—biologically, at least. A significant number of women experience early menopause, with up to 8.6% entering "premature" menopause before the age of 40 (Choe & Sung, 2020). This realization can bring a mix of amazement and alarm. The lesson here? Expect the unexpected—and perhaps carry a fan, just in case.

Myth #2: Menopause Is the Same for Everyone

Have you ever wondered why, when you're chatting with your friends about symptoms, some have no clue what you're talking about? Well, that's because no two menopause experiences are alike. Your hot flash could be your friend's night sweats. Why is this important? Because these differences highlight the crucial understanding that everyone's journey is personal and unique. Much like orders at a coffee shop, menopause comes in several forms—none quite the same as the others. Some women sail through it smoothly, while others hit choppy waters. This variability stems from individual health, genetics, and lifestyle factors. It's as if life is giving you a secret menu you didn't ask for, filled with surprises—some delightful, some not so much.

Myth #3: Menopause Kills Your Sex Drive

Sometimes, it feels like Mother Nature decided to throw a surprise party but forgot to invite your sex drive to the festivities. Let's address the myth that menopause "kills" your sex drive.

First off, menopause might change your body's game a bit, but it doesn't necessarily mean the end of your libido. It's more like that surprising development in a rom-com—unexpected but not necessarily bad! Some women might find that hormonal changes lead to decreased libido, while others might experience a new sense of freedom, realizing they don't have to worry about unintended pregnancies anymore. Talk about a silver lining!

While menopause might bring some dry spells (pun intended), it can also lead to creative solutions, such as experimenting with different forms of intimacy or trying out new activities together (more to come later). So, rather than seeing menopause as the Grim Reaper of your sex life, think of it as an opportunity to explore uncharted territories!

Scientific Realities

Understanding menopause from a scientific perspective helps demystify this often misunderstood transition. Science tells us that menopause isn't merely an ending; it's a biological milestone marking new beginnings. This revelation frees us from the myths that label menopause as something negative, and instead, it empowers us to embrace the future with hope and optimism.

However, society loves a good stereotype. We've all heard "menopausal" used pejoratively, suggesting irrationality or emotional instability. Such narratives make menopause sound like a bad running joke that everyone laughs at awkwardly. But why laugh when we can educate and empower? Breaking free from these labels elevates our collective understanding while challenging societal misconceptions and allows women to reclaim control over how they're perceived during menopause. Remember, menopause isn't synonymous with losing purpose; on the contrary, it paves the way for self-discovery and newfound strength. Post-menopause, women contribute in vibrant ways to their families and communities, illustrating their continued relevance and value.

Instead of stigmatizing menopause, let's change its narrative. When someone dismisses symptoms like mood swings or forgetfulness as simply being "hormonal," it diminishes the very real impacts of menopause. Recognizing these symptoms creates empathy rather than ridicule, leading society toward inclusivity instead of exclusion. Encouraging open conversations disarms stigma, normalizing menopause as part of the universal human experience.

Why Humor Matters in Managing Menopause

Menopause can feel like a roller-coaster ride, but what if laughter could be your seat belt? Humor can be a powerful ally during menopause, offering relief from stress and restoring a sense of perspective.

The Healing Power of Laughter

Let's start by exploring how humor acts as a therapeutic tool. During menopause, stress levels can skyrocket because of hormonal fluctuations. This stress manifests, among other ways, in increased levels of hormones such as epinephrine and cortisol. However, laughter can come to the rescue as a natural stress reliever. Studies have shown that genuine laughter reduces cortisol levels: When you chuckle, your body releases endorphins, which foster a sense of well-being and relaxation (Youngblood Gregory, 2024).

"Menopause: the time in a woman's life where 'Are you hot?' is no longer a pick-up line." – Anonymous

Laughter is often said to be the best medicine, and when it comes to menopause, it might just be the secret ingredient to surviving the chaos. Responding to those hot flashes and hormone swings with a side of belly laughs sounds like a recipe for resilience. As well as relieving tension, laughter recharges your mood and gives a cheeky wink to your challenges.

Handling tough conversations? Humor is your trusty sidekick, helping to soften the edges of challenging topics. "I feel like a werewolf from a romantic comedy!" is much more relatable—and less daunting—than "I'm struggling with all these chin hairs!" Using humor can make it easier to articulate your feelings, opening the door for more genuine communication without the heavy baggage.

So, embrace laughter as part of your menopause survival kit! It may not cure everything, but it's undoubtedly an essential supporter. Inject humor into life; even menopause can be funny.

Comedic Coping Strategies

Take laughter yoga, for example, which combines forced laughter with breathing techniques. It's a playful yet practical approach to reducing stress and improving mood. While it might seem unconventional, this practice enhances optimism and decreases depression, proving that even intentional laughter carries significant psychological benefits.

Why not consider keeping a humor journal? Documenting funny incidents or reflections will capture the joyful moments and provide a resource for uplifting your spirits when facing menopausal blues. Create a habit of looking at life through a lighter lens, building resilience against the stressors inherent to menopause. It can be compared to working out a particular muscle—the harder you use it, the stronger it becomes.

Laughter is a potent force; it doesn't just reduce stress hormones, it also offers cardiovascular benefits by improving blood flow and enhancing vessel function. So, while you're giggling away, your heart gets a workout too! Plus, laughter encourages muscle relaxation and improved respiratory function, thanks to the deep breathing it involves. It's a full-body mini-rejuvenation session every time you crack a smile.

Incorporating laughter doesn't mean we're ignoring the challenges of menopause; instead, we're facing them with a refreshed perspective. This can help you position yourself to handle menopause with stronger coping skills. Challenges become more manageable, less overwhelming, and more surmountable when viewed through laughter.

Think about the last good laugh you had. How did it make you feel? The joy that follows laughter is infectious and transformative.

It can turn even the most stressful day into one filled with warmth and companionship. Embrace it as part of your menopausal journey; you'll likely find the road a bit smoother and the burdens lighter.

Why Talking About Menopause Matters

Talking about menopause can feel as uncomfortable as wearing wool socks in summer. However, it's time to kick the hush-hush habit to the curb and bring menopause into the open. For many women, menopause isn't just a phase but a transformation. By discussing this natural stage, we begin to dismantle the stigma that often shrouds it. Openly discussing menopause, like acne or puberty, normalizes it. Not talking about menopause is like ignoring an elephant trying to squeeze through a dog door—incredibly awkward and, in fact, impossible.

When we're educated about what our bodies are going through, we gain control over our experiences, empowering ourselves to make better choices for our health and well-being. Knowing what to expect means fewer surprises during those hot flashes at the grocery store.

Linda's Laughter Journey

Meet Linda, a woman in her fabulous 50s who suddenly found herself on the unexpected wild ride of menopause. One minute, she was enjoying her morning coffee; the next, she was soaked in sweat like she'd just run a marathon in a sauna. Nothing says "good morning" quite like that feeling of being a human slip-and-slide!

As if that weren't enough, Linda began to notice unwanted chin hair sprouting like weeds. Armed with tweezers, she felt like she was on a never-ending quest to battle her facial fur. "I didn't sign up for this—where's my fairy godmother to grant me a hair-free wish?" she joked to herself, hoping for magical help.

Then, the brain fog made her forget whether she'd left the oven on or was even supposed to be cooking. One day, while discussing dinner plans with her husband, she suddenly discussed the merits of becoming a professional cat whisperer. Where did that come from? Who knew what was going on in her mind? All she could do was laugh at how lost she felt.

The most comical part of all was her reaction to commercial breaks. Linda realized she'd developed an affinity for cat commercials, and she found herself tearing up at every adopt-a-cat ad. "Who knew Mr. Whiskers could tug at my heartstrings this much?" she laughed, realizing she was crying as if she'd just watched a heart-wrenching drama.

As the days turned into weeks, Linda started embracing her menopausal symptoms with humor. She spent time with friends, laughing until they cried while bonding over their shared experiences.

She also created a mantra— Sweat is just the body's way of making you feel alive!"—and began celebrating those soaked sheets as badges of honor rather than sources of frustration. The brain fog? She started calling it her "creative enhancement period," where new and ridiculous ideas were endless, even if they didn't always make sense.

Linda soon discovered that laughter was her superpower. The more she leaned into humor, the easier it became to handle her symptoms. No longer a prisoner to embarrassment or frustration, she took the wheel back in her unexpected journey. With every laugh, she found connection, relief, and the realization that she wasn't alone in this experience.

And so, with her (slightly furry) chin held high, Linda became the comedic queen of menopause, sharing her stories and making light of her experiences. After all, when life gives you lemons (or chin hairs), you could turn them into a comedy show!

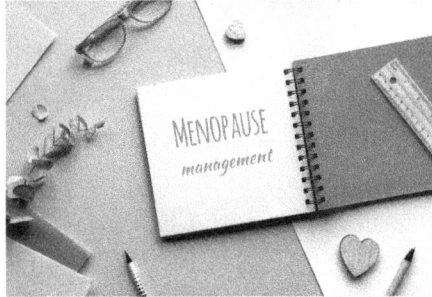

Breaking the Menopause Silence in the Workplace

In workplaces, breaking the silence on menopause can cause significant change. Many women still feel the sting of stigma at work, leading to quiet suffering that affects their performance. A 2024 study reports that 72% of women have hidden their menopausal symptoms at least once in their workplace (Catalyst, 2024). When organizations refuse to acknowledge and address health matters, such as menopause, they risk losing talented employees. Employers must raise awareness and provide support systems that allow women to be open about their symptoms without fear of prejudice.

Menopause isn't something that should be whispered about behind closed doors. Talking about it openly can lead to greater understanding and acceptance, helping ease the metaphorical weight of carrying secrets. According to health experts, recognizing menopause as a normal aspect of life—as natural as the changing seasons—can significantly improve our quality of life (Aninye et al., 2021). Too often, it's treated as a deficiency, but embracing it instead can lead to empowerment and preparation for life beyond menopause.

Bringing It All Together

As you journey through menopause, embracing laughter and understanding can make all the difference. We've explored how humor is more than just a giggle; it's your trusty companion for handling the ups and downs of this natural transition. Seeing menopause from a humorous perspective brightens your days and opens doors to meaningful discussions. Laughter lightens the load, inviting conversations, breaking taboos, and promoting empathy. Every shared chuckle helps build connections with those who understand what you're going through, transforming potentially lonely moments into opportunities for growth and sisterhood.

When you tackle menopause with an open mind and a playful heart, you inspire yourself to challenge misconceptions and reclaim control over this stage of life. Understanding your body during menopause is like trying to assemble IKEA furniture without the instructions—it's confusing, a bit overwhelming, and there's always one piece you can't find. But fear not! Understanding menopause improves decision-making and self-awareness.

While menopause might present you with a plate full of challenges, it also offers heaps of self-discovery and newfound strength. So, go ahead and laugh at the absurdity of it all—making this time uniquely yours means turning hormonal hijinks into a comedy special starring you!

Let's jump into the next chapter (trying not to work up a sweat), where we'll examine the science behind menopause. It's time to figure out why our bodies feel like they're turning on us!

Chapter Two

What the Heck Is Happening to My Body?

E xplaining menopause is like trying to solve a Rubik's Cube while riding a bucking bronco. It is exciting, but it can feel a tad impossible! On the surface, it's just hormones hosting a wild party in your body, but scratch that glittery surface, and you'll see it's a twisted soap opera.

Menopause isn't the finale; it's the ultimate "glow-up" challenge that comes after decades of life. Just as autumn leaves strut their vibrant colors, women entering menopause get to flaunt their dazzling transformations. These are often surprising, sometimes bizarre, but always worthy of a round of applause. Hold tight as we embark on this hormonal ups and downs ride, discovering what each twist and turn means for your body and brain!

"Menopause is just puberty's evil older sister."–Anonymous

If you are like me, your mother never told you about menopause, or should I say, "warned"! Understanding is half the battle, and that starts with estrogen, and follows its dramatic entrances and exits, which can swing your energy level from that of a caffeinated squirrel to a sleepy sloth.

We will also explore physical issues like night sweats and vaginal dryness, all while maintaining a light and humorous tone, because after all, laughter is the best medicine, right? Ultimately, this chapter is your map to understanding and equipping yourself during this epic adventure.

Hormonal Fluctuations and Their Effects

Understanding what's happening during this phase of your life can help you stay in control, even when it feels as if your hormones have jumped on a skateboard and forgotten to invite your sense of calm.

HORMONE QUICK REFERENCE:
Estrogen: Affects 200+ body systems
Progesterone: The "calming hormone"
Testosterone: Desire, energy, muscle
Impact: All decline during menopause

The Dramatic Drop in Estrogen

Estrogen takes center stage in this hormonal drama. It's the hormone responsible for more bodily functions than it seems fair to pin on one molecule. As menopause approaches, typically in a woman's late 40s to early 50s, estrogen production begins its slow waltz out the door. This decrease isn't always subtle, either. It's a bit like when your favorite band decides to break up suddenly—unexpected and not ideal.

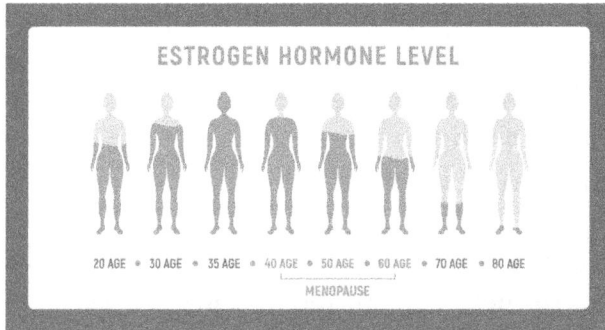

ESTROGEN HORMONE LEVEL

20 AGE • 30 AGE • 35 AGE • 40 AGE • 50 AGE • 60 AGE • 70 AGE • 80 AGE

MENOPAUSE

Hormonal fluctuations during menopause can feel as if you're on a runaway bumper car with no brakes—terrifying and unpredictable! As estrogen levels begin to drop, the ride intensifies, causing a cascade of symptoms that can leave women wondering if they've accidentally joined a thrill-seeker's adventure.

Physical Symptoms

- **Hot flashes** are your own personal summer, coming just when you least expect them, turning you into a human sauna.

- Then there are **night sweats**; it's as if your body's decided to have a mid sleep pool party.

- **Vaginal dryness** adds its awkward touch to the mix, making intimacy feel more like a desert expedition than a romantic rendezvous.

- **Irregular periods** are the wild card, playing hide-and-seek without hinting when they'll appear next.

- And speaking of **sleep**, those solid eight hours are now just a dream. Whether you're being woken by sweat or needing to pee, exhaustion is your new best friend.

- Welcome also to **joint and muscle pain**, which makes you feel like you've taken up a new hobby: amateur wrestling.

- Your **skin** morphs into a parchment-like canvas perfect for a Renaissance painting.

- **Weight gain** usually loves to camp out in the belly area, as if it's the new hangout spot in town.

- **Reduced bone density** makes you appreciate those high school track workouts, as that early impact exercise helped build bone strength that offers some protection to you now.

Emotional and Cognitive Symptoms

- **Mood swings** might toss you around like a weather vane in a storm. One minute, you're laughing; the next, you're crying over a cute animal video.

- **Anxiety and depression** can crash the party, leaving you feeling like a moody teenager again.

- Add **low energy levels**, and getting off the couch requires a motivational speech.

- **Brain fog** can turn even simple tasks into challenging brain teasers.

- **Reduced libido** might mean romance feels less appealing than a slice of cold pizza.

- **Headaches or migraines** can become frequent visitors.

- **Urinary symptoms** may keep you on a first-name basis with every bathroom within a mile radius.

- **Changes in breast tissue** add another unpredictable twist.

Recognizing these signs of hormonal shifts isn't just a part of riding the menopausal roller coaster; it's key to proactive symptom management. Understanding why emotions can swing like a pendulum when estrogen dips can help you tackle those difficulties with a little more grace and a lot more humor!

Progesterone: The Unsung Hero of Menstrual Cycles

First, we need to give progesterone the standing ovation it deserves. Progesterone is the stage manager of your menstrual cycle. It's not flashy, but it's essential for the show to run smoothly. Produced primarily by the ovaries following ovulation, progesterone prepares the uterus for potential pregnancy by thickening its lining. If pregnancy doesn't occur, progesterone levels drop, and the curtain rises on your period.

The Sleep Saga: Progesterone and Insomnia

Lower levels of progesterone can wreak havoc on your sleep patterns. Remember those nights when you could fall asleep as soon as your head hit the pillow? Well, progesterone was partly responsible for that. This hormone has a calming effect, acting like a natural sedative. When levels drop, insomnia can become an issue. Understanding this connection can enable you to have productive conversations with your doctor about treatment options, such as bioidentical hormones or lifestyle changes, to reclaim your rest.

Menopause isn't a malfunction; it's a transition. Knowing how progesterone works, and what happens when it doesn't, helps normalize this stage of life. Armed with this knowledge, you can confidently tackle these changes, with your doctor, your sleep playlist, and perhaps a hefty dose of melatonin.

Testosterone Levels: The Quiet Contender in Menopause

Testosterone—the "forgotten" hormone of menopause—deserves attention. While it's more famous for its starring role in male biology, testosterone is just as vital for women. During menopause, levels of this hormone can dip dramatically for some women, leading to a slew of symptoms that can leave you feeling a little less... you.

Here are the symptoms of testosterone decline:

- **Decreased muscle mass:** If the gym suddenly feels like an Olympic event, you're not imagining it. Testosterone helps maintain muscle tone, so lower levels can lead to loss of strength and definition.

- **Increased fatigue:** Feeling tired just walking to the fridge? Reduced testosterone levels can zap your stamina.

- **Reduced sexual sensation and orgasmic difficulty:** Sensitivity and arousal can decrease, making sexual enjoyment and satisfaction a distant memory. While these symptoms can make intimacy challenging, they're not insurmountable. Open communication with your partner and healthcare provider can lead to solutions, from hormonal treatments to lubricants.

- **Lack of motivation:** Ever feel like hitting the couch is a bigger accomplishment than hitting the gym? That's the motivation drain in action.

- **Increased stress levels:** Hormonal changes make your stress radar hypersensitive.

- **Reduced energy levels:** Maintaining momentum

throughout the day feels like running a marathon—without the medal.

- **Changes in physical endurance:** Climbing stairs or carrying groceries may feel more challenging as your stamina wanes.

Awareness of testosterone's role can also help you make lifestyle adjustments—starting to do strength training or making dietary changes, for instance—to mitigate the impact.

Hormonal Interactions: A Complex Symphony

Hormones don't work in isolation; they're like your body's orchestra, with each one playing a vital part in the grand symphony of your health. The whole piece can feel off-key when one section (maybe progesterone or testosterone) goes out of tune. Enter the domino effect:

- Lower estrogen can exacerbate symptoms of low testosterone, such as reduced libido and energy levels.

- Decreased progesterone might intensify sleep disturbances, compounding the fatigue from low testosterone.

- Cortisol, the stress hormone, often skyrockets during this time, further draining your energy and disrupting hormonal harmony.

Treatments might include HRT, stress management techniques, and exercise routines tailored to your needs. We'll explore all of these in the upcoming chapters.

Menopause may feel like a hormonal game of Jenga, but knowledge is your cheat sheet. By understanding the roles of progesterone and testosterone and their intricate interplay, you can advocate for yourself, normalize this transition, and embrace the changes with a healthy dose of humor—and maybe a glass of wine. (Red wine contains antioxidants, after all ...)

Michelle's Midlife Hormonal Circus

Meet Michelle, 48, who stars in her personal reality show, *Hormones Gone Wild*. Until a year ago, she felt pretty in tune with her body—exercising, eating well, and enjoying a decent night's sleep. Then menopause barged in like an uninvited houseguest, bringing insomnia, mood swings, and a libido that went on sabbatical.

It started when she blanked during a work presentation—unusual for her sharp mind. Later that night, wide awake at 3:00 a.m., she wondered, *What's happening to me?* A little research led her to discover that low progesterone levels were likely behind her insomnia. Progesterone, the calming hormone, had left the building. Armed with this knowledge, Michelle saw her doctor, who suggested bioidentical progesterone cream. Slowly, her sleep and focus improved.

Meanwhile, Michelle noticed other changes. Her legs felt weak during yoga, shopping bags seemed heavier, and her energy was nonexistent. Libido? Forget about it. She felt disconnected, not just from her husband, Dan, but also from herself. Another chat with her doctor revealed that low testosterone was affecting her energy, muscle tone, and desire for intimacy. The solution? Weight training, stress management, and protein-packed meals helped her start feeling stronger and more vibrant.

One rough morning after snapping at Dan, Michelle realized *she couldn't control her hormones, but she could control how she responded.* She began journaling her symptoms and moods, noticing patterns:

stress made everything worse, and exercise made her feel better. She also opened up to Dan, saying, "It's not you; it's my hormones." They worked together to reconnect, trying lubricants, planning date nights, and cutting each other some slack.

Now, a year into her menopause journey, Michelle still has tough days but doesn't let them define her. Weight lifting has brought back her strength. Her sleep is better, and her relationship with Dan is stronger. "Menopause isn't the end of the world. It's just a plot twist," she says, raising her glass to herself and every woman rewriting her story.

The Stages: Perimenopause to Post-menopause

Each menopause stage is a unique chapter, unfolding its challenges and revelatory insights. Accepting this involves understanding each phase—perimenopause, menopause, and post-menopause—and their distinctive characteristics.

Stage One: Perimenopause

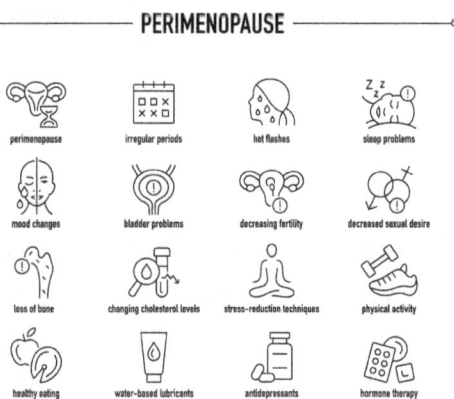

PERIMENOPAUSE

perimenopause · irregular periods · hot flashes · sleep problems

mood changes · bladder problems · decreasing fertility · decreased sexual desire

loss of bone · changing cholesterol levels · stress-reduction techniques · physical activity

healthy eating · water-based lubricants · antidepressants · hormone therapy

Perimenopause presents with subtle signals that may initially seem like random disturbances in life's rhythm. Consider it the opening act of menopause, with fluctuating hormones setting the stage for the changes to come. During perimenopause, your body begins to experience irregular menstrual cycles and unpredictable hormone levels. These fluctuations are life's little reminders that change is the only constant. You might experience hot flashes, mood swings, and even sleep disruptions that inspire impromptu midnight musings. As these symptoms wax and wane, it's essential to approach them with curiosity and patience.

Perimenopause invites you to glide and adapt to its variable tempo like learning a new dance. This period can span several years, making it important to understand that while the road may occasionally be bumpy, it's leading you toward a new chapter of life.

Stage Two: Menopause

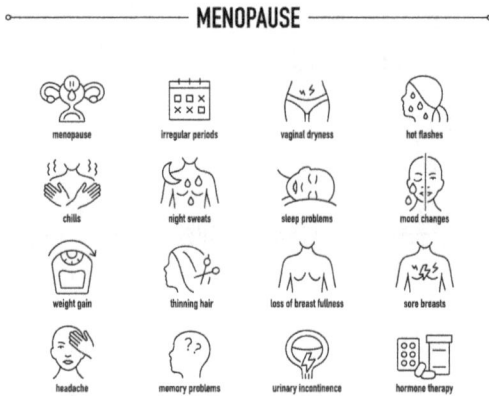

Next, we reach menopause itself. Officially, doctors diagnose menopause after a woman has gone 12 consecutive months without a menstrual period (NHS Inform, 2024). So, if you haven't had your "friend" for 10 months, and she pays you a visit in month 11, you start over. Yup, even I was shocked to find that out!

Think of menopause as a rite of passage, signaling the conclusion of your reproductive years. It's a time that brings about closure but may also require some emotional adjustment. Many women find themselves confronting mixed emotions; there's no one-size-fits-all response. For some, menopause feels liberating, offering freedom from monthly cycles and concerns about pregnancy. For others, it might bring nostalgia for life's earlier phases or anxiety about bodily changes and aging. Owning your feelings allows you to embrace this life stage fully, recognizing menopause as a conclusion to one phase of your life and the start of a new era filled with possibilities.

The Finale: Post-menopause

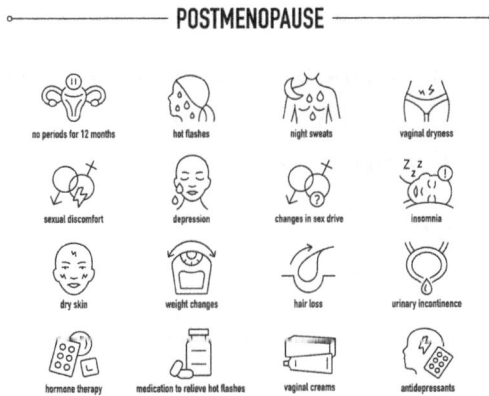

Post-menopause follows, bringing a fresh set of challenging and empowering considerations. As the curtain rises on this stage, many previous symptoms may gradually recede, offering a semblance of peace after the turmoil that came before.

However, it's a time to pay attention to new health risks that become more pronounced due to changing hormone levels, such as osteoporosis. Emphasizing bone health through diet, exercise, and regular medical checkups becomes vital in safeguarding your well-being. In this phase, your health isn't just about managing symptoms but proactively nurturing longevity and strength. It's an opportunity to redefine wellness on your terms, focusing on personal growth and self-discovery.

Transition Variability

Within these stages lies the kaleidoscope of transition variability—a reminder that menopause is an intensely personal journey. Every woman's experience is unique, shaped by individual circumstances and biology. This diversity calls for empathy and understanding, sharing our stories, and building supportive communities. By connecting with others on similar journeys, we gain strength in numbers and wisdom from our collective experiences. There's power in personalization; strategies that work brilliantly for one person may need fine-tuning for another. Thus, forging a path that resonates with your unique needs is paramount. It's time to listen to your body and respect its signals, allowing you to change menopause from a silent struggle into a motivating dialogue.

As you move through the stages of menopause, remember this overarching theme: Each phase is not an isolated silo but part of a broader narrative of feminine resilience and evolution. The variations in our experiences remind us of our individuality while underscoring our shared humanity.

Reflecting upon the changes, we discover that laughter, acceptance, and adaptability are our friends. Humor, in particular, proves invaluable; it lightens the journey and offers perspective when things feel overwhelming.

The Changes Keep Coming

Understanding menopause involves grasping the many physical changes that can occur as your body passes through this natural phase of life. It's doesn't just involve hot flashes and mood swings. There are several significant health considerations to keep in mind, particularly regarding your bones, heart, metabolism, and muscle mass.

Bone Health

First on the list is bone health. During menopause, your estrogen levels drop, which might make your bones as fragile as a house of cards. Hormonal changes are directly tied to decreases in bone density, escalating the risk of osteoporosis—a condition where bones become weak and brittle, leaving them susceptible to fractures. It's like trying to balance on ice wearing roller skates; without strong bones as your safety net, you're at greater risk for injuries.

Let me geek out a little here and explain estrogen. Your body makes three main types of estrogen that do different jobs throughout your life:

Estradiol (E2)
This is the strongest type of estrogen and the most common one during your reproductive years. It helps control your menstrual cycle and keeps your bones strong. When you reach menopause, estradiol levels drop significantly, which can cause hot flashes and make your bones more fragile.

Estrone (E1)
After menopause, this becomes your main estrogen. It's weaker than estradiol and is made from fat tissue in your body. Some research suggests that elevated estrone levels may be associated with increased health risks in certain populations; discuss your individual risk factors with your healthcare provider.

Estriol (E3)
This is the weakest form of estrogen and only shows up in large amounts during pregnancy. It helps support the growing baby and prepares your body for childbirth.

As you go through different life stages, these three estrogens shift in importance; from the strong estradiol during your younger years, to mostly estrone after menopause, with estriol playing its special role during pregnancy.

What's A Girl To Do?

Fear not, for there's a saving grace: weight-bearing exercises and vitamin D intake. Regular activities such as walking, jogging, or strength training can help maintain bone density—and don't forget to get enough calcium and vitamin D (Holland, 2024). Think of these nutrients as the glue that keeps your skeletal system intact. Calcium can be found in dairy products and leafy greens like kale and broccoli, while vitamin D is something you can soak up from the sun. Start eating fatty fish about three times a week—salmon or mackerel are great choices—as well as milk and some cereals because they're great sources of vitamin D from food. Check out the Bonuses after the Conclusion that detail sources of calcium and vitamin D.

Heart Health

Menopause not only impacts bone health but also heightens the risk to heart health. With the significant decline in estradiol (E2), the most potent form of estrogen during reproductive years, women face an increased risk of cardiovascular issues after menopause (Williamson, 2023). Much like your high school sweetheart, your heart needs attention and care, especially during these years.

Menopause significantly influences cardiovascular health, leading to an increased risk of heart attacks in women. Here's an overview of the statistics and contributing factors:

Statistics

- **Increased Incidence Post-Menopause:** The Framingham Heart Study reported a 2.6-fold higher incidence of cardiovascular events in postmenopausal women compared to premenopausal counterparts of the same age. (Kostis & Wilson, 2020)

- **Age-Related Risk:** Women develop cardiovascular diseases (CVD) on average 7–10 years later than men, primarily because of estrogen's protective effects. However, this advantage diminishes after menopause, leading to a rise in heart disease cases among older women.

- **Prevalence:** Over 60 million women (44%) in the United States are living with some form of heart disease. Causes and contributing factors include:

1. **Estrogen Decline:** Estrogen helps keep blood vessels relaxed and open. With less estrogen during menopause, cholesterol may build up on artery walls, increasing the risk of heart disease or stroke.

2. **Adverse Changes in Cardiovascular Risk Factors:**

   ○ **Lipid Profile:** Postmenopausal women often experience higher levels of total cholesterol, triglycerides, and low-density lipoprotein (LDL-C), along with reduced high-density lipoprotein (HDL-C) levels.

   ○ **Blood Pressure:** The hormonal changes that occur during menopause can bring increased cardiovascular risk as higher blood pressure.

3. **Weight Gain and Fat Distribution:** Menopause can lead to weight gain, especially around the waist, which is associated with a higher risk of heart disease.

4. **Early Menopause:** Women experiencing menopause before the age of 45 have a higher risk of coronary heart disease, likely because of a longer duration without estrogen's protective effects.

5. **Lifestyle Factors:** During menopause, factors such as increased blood pressure, cholesterol levels, and weight gain can elevate the risk of heart disease.

6. **Psychosocial Factors:** Depression and sleep disturbances during menopause have been linked to an increased risk of heart disease.

It's important to take action. Emphasizing lifestyle modifications, such as maintaining a balanced diet low in saturated fats and rich in fruits and vegetables, is increasingly important. Regular aerobic exercise, such as swimming or dancing, can also do wonders for your cardiovascular system by improving circulation and reducing blood pressure. And don't underestimate the power of open discussions with your healthcare provider. Regular checkups and honest conversations about heart health can prevent many potential issues.

Bringing It All Together

Understanding the whirlwind of biological and hormonal changes during menopause is much like trying to befriend a tornado; it's chaotic. Still, you can find calm in the storm with the right approach. This chapter moved through the dramatic exit of estrogen, progesterone, and testosterone, bringing along brain fog, bone loss, and unexpected challenges. Acknowledging these shifts empowers you to take control rather than letting them rule your world. Remember, you're not alone on this roller coaster. From lifestyle tweaks, such as choosing your diet wisely, to considering medical interventions and supplements, various paths exist to manage this phase more easily and comfortably.

As menopause unfolds, it invites reflection on this profound transition in life. Whether perimenopause sneaks in or post-menopause offers a new perspective, understanding these stages allows for a personalized approach to managing your symptoms. Embrace humor and patience as your companions; they help lighten the heavier moments and transform them into opportunities for growth and empowerment. Let this time serve as a reminder of female resilience and adaptability.

You're now equipped with the knowledge and strategies to change the overwhelming ride of menopause into an adventure filled with strength and self-discovery. It's time to move into the next chapter, where we'll discover real, usable tips and tricks to get through menopause symptoms with ease and laughter.

Chapter Three

Hot Flash? Meet Your Match

S potting symptoms and acting against them is like trying to control a wayward garden hose. Things might get messy, yet you're determined to wrestle it back into order without drenching yourself in the process. As you start this adventure, be prepared for a trip through a landscape filled with those delightful gifts of menopause—night sweats and brain fog—that materialize out of nowhere, livening up your day or night.

Even as they rudely crash the party of your otherwise well-ordered life, there's power in understanding their antics. After all, forewarned is forearmed! With plenty of laughs and a dollop of insight, we'll untangle the chaos these symptoms bring into our lives and give them a run for their money.

In this chapter, we'll examine the art of managing these pesky symptoms with grace and ingenuity. From identifying what sets them off, which might include everything from spicy foods to stress, to understanding why on Earth your body's temperature control has gone AWOL, we'll decipher every twist and turn of these experiences. Take a breath and remind yourself that you've got tools, humor, and time on your side.

Hot Flashes and Night Sweats

Hot flashes, those unexpected bursts of warmth that feel like standing before a roaring fire at the most inconvenient times, are a hallmark of menopause. They begin as a sudden wave of heat rising through your body, usually followed by redness and sweating. It runs its course, and you're along for the ride.

These episodes can last for mere seconds to several minutes, causing discomfort, panic, anxiety, and sometimes embarrassment in social situations. Understanding what's happening physiologically during a hot flash can illuminate these moments.

Physiologically, hot flashes occur due to changes in your body's thermostat, primarily influenced by fluctuating hormone levels. The biggest culprit? Estrogen! The reduced sensitivity of the hypothalamus—the part of your brain that regulates body temperature—leads to these sudden thermal events. Think of it as your internal thermostat mistaking a comfortably warm room for a sauna and triggering mechanisms to cool you down, including expanding blood vessels and activating sweat glands. These physical responses result in a hot flash's familiar flush and moisture. Understanding these changes can help you better manage and cope with your symptoms (Goins, 2023).

Night sweats are the nocturnal wicked stepmothers of hot flashes, making their grand entrance when you're least prepared to deal with them—in the middle of sleep. Characterized by excessive sweating during the night, they often awaken you from slumber, leaving your sheets and pajamas drenched and your sleep disrupted. The aftermath of such interruptions can affect your mood, cognitive function, and overall health, turning restful nights into exhausting ones.

How to Cope Without Losing Your Mind

Effective management of night sweats and hot flashes begins with understanding their triggers. Common culprits include:

- stress

- spicy foods

- caffeine

- alcohol

- environmental heat

When you can pinpoint your personal triggers, you gain a way to manage the frequency and intensity of your symptoms. For instance, reducing your caffeine intake throughout the day or avoiding a hot shower right before bed might help mitigate nighttime disturbances (Goins, 2023).

How do you figure out your triggers? Journal! Yep, start jotting it down each day when you've had a hot flash or night sweats. Ask yourself questions like, "Did I eat something different?" or "Was I more stressed than usual?" Pay attention to the amount of caffeine you had or if you had wine with dinner. After a few weeks, review your notes and see what patterns appear. You should get a clear picture of what triggers your internal combustion. Additionally, consider consulting a healthcare professional to help you identify and manage your triggers effectively.

Incorporate Cooling Tools

Adjust your routine to incorporate cooling tools designed to combat these vasomotor symptoms. In other words, get yourself some fans. I have a small one blowing directly in my face while I sleep and one on my desk while I work. Oh, did I mention the mini one I carry in my purse for those grocery store lineups and the "Oh my, it's a thousand degrees in this car!" moments? Being prepared with these tools can make a world of difference.

It's also super important to start dressing in layers. Then, when you feel those heat waves coming on, you can always remove a light sweater if you have a T-shirt underneath, right?

Now, let's chat about breathable fabrics because they can make a world of difference. I didn't even know what bamboo fabric was until my wise (already through menopause) aunt bought me a pair of pajamas made from it. Even when you wake up swimming in your own juices, this material, somehow, stays dry. They even make bedsheets with it. Get some!

Cooling pillows are another must. If you haven't heard of these, you're welcome. They aim to keep your head and face cool while sleeping. You can find them on Amazon and at most home goods stores.

Creating a comfortable sleep environment involves keeping your bedroom well-ventilated (my window stays open even in winter) and maintaining a cooler room temperature. This approach not only helps combat night sweats but also promotes better-quality sleep overall, making you feel cared for and comfortable.

Finally, I will let you know one of my all-time best-kept secrets. Beside my bed is what I call a "nighttime chill kit." I picked out a pretty basket, and inside put a dry pillowcase, new jammies and underwear, a cooling body spray, cooling wipes, and a bottle of water. Before I go to bed each night, I also toss in a new ice pack. I started doing this because I was tired of waking up overheated, soaked, and exhausted. I would fumble around in the dark, trying to find clean, dry clothing without waking my hubby. Now, everything I need is beside me, and I barely have to wake up to get it.

Bring on the Relaxation and Lifestyle Choices

Relaxation techniques can also be great friends during menopause. Stress is a known exacerbator of hot flashes and night sweats, so incorporating deep breathing, meditation, or yoga into your daily routine can be helpful. These activities help lower stress levels and may reduce the severity and frequency of vasomotor symptoms over time. A few minutes of mindfulness before bed could lead to fewer nighttime disruptions and more restorative rest (Bianchi et al., 2016).

Don't agonize too much about this. I know we can read the word "mindfulness" and get images of being twisted up like a pretzel with sounding bowls all around the room. But it can be as simple as you need it to be. There are plenty of mindfulness apps you can download. Alternative, just, sit quietly for a minute, inhale through your nose for four counts, then exhale through your mouth for four counts. Repeat three times, and voilà, welcome to mindfulness.

Here are three highly-rated mindfulness apps known for their effectiveness, user experience, and positive reviews (at the time of this writing). Search for them and see which might work for you.

1. Headspace

2. Calm

3. Insight Timer

While self-care strategies help when managing these symptoms, it's important to acknowledge the power of lifestyle choices. It's time to kick that smoking habit and maintain a balanced diet because both can indirectly influence your body's response to menopausal symptoms. Meanwhile, regular physical activity boosts your mood and physical health and helps you regulate your body temperature more effectively.

Real Talk: If you can't take it any longer and hot flashes are interfering with your life, you might need to consider medical intervention, especially if self-management proves insufficient. HRT can offer relief by balancing your hormones and alleviating some of your menopausal symptoms. However, it's essential to consult a healthcare provider to weigh the benefits and risks specific to your health profile. Alternatively, medications such as certain SSRIs (selective serotonin reuptake inhibitor) have been shown to help alleviate vasomotor symptoms for some women and could be an option to explore under professional guidance (Goins, 2023).

An SSRI is a type of antidepressant medication commonly used to treat depression, anxiety disorders, panic disorders, and certain other mental health conditions.

How SSRIs Work

- Serotonin's Role: Serotonin is a neurotransmitter that contributes to feelings of well-being and happiness.

- Mechanism: SSRIs work by blocking the reabsorption (reuptake) of serotonin into neurons, increasing the amount of serotonin available in the brain. This helps improve mood and reduce anxiety.

Managing Sleep Disturbances

Sleep! That elusive friend women in menopause yearn to welcome back into their nightly routines. If you're tossing and turning at night, rest assured you're not alone. Menopause can be tricky when it comes to catching quality zzzs, thanks to the hormonal changes that ride shotgun with the transition. These shifts often lead to disrupted sleep cycles, making you feel like you've suddenly signed up for an unintended nocturnal lifestyle.

So, why is this happening? It all boils down to the estrogen and progesterone upheaval we discussed in the previous chapter. These hormones influence your body's temperature regulation and consequently affect your sleep-wake cycle. When they decide to dip and dive, you're left dealing with symptoms such as hot flashes and night sweats, which can rudely awaken you from a deep slumber. Managing these interruptions calls for a strong strategy. But how? Try these tricks:

- **Sleep hygiene:** I know "hygiene" might make you think of brushing your teeth or washing your hands, but sleep hygiene encompasses habits that help you fall asleep and stay asleep more effectively. Let's start with something simple yet vital: a bedtime routine. This isn't just for kids who need a story before shutting their eyes; adults benefit greatly, too. By sticking to a consistent sleep schedule—going to bed and waking up at the same time every day—you teach your body to set its internal clock. This simple practice can improve your sleep quality.

- **Create a sanctuary:** It's time to create a restful sleeping environment! Consider your bedroom a retreat. Keep it cool, dark, and quiet, and if external disturbances are your nemesis, invest in blackout curtains or a white noise machine.

- **Banish those screens:** The blue light emitted by phones and tablets can mess with your melatonin levels, the hormone responsible for making you sleepy. Try winding down with a book instead. Remember, your bedroom should whisper "rest," not "work" or "play."

- **Watch what you drink:** There's also the question of what to sip. Caffeine lovers, pay attention: Swap out those evening coffees for soothing herbal teas. And remember, alcohol may get you snoozy, but it ultimately disrupts sleep later in the night.

My weakness is carbonated drinks, which can make you pee more, but the reason depends on the specific type of drink:

1. Caffeinated Carbonated Drinks (e.g., Cola, Energy Drinks)

- Caffeine as a Diuretic: Caffeine increases urine production by stimulating the kidneys to release more water. This can lead to more frequent urination.

- Higher Risk with Excessive Caffeine: Drinking large amounts of caffeinated sodas or energy drinks can enhance this effect.

2. Carbonated Water (e.g., Sparkling Water, Seltzer)

- Mild Effect: Plain carbonated water itself is not a diuretic. However, the increased fluid intake can naturally lead to more frequent urination.

- Bladder Irritation: For some individuals, the carbonation can irritate the bladder lining, leading to a sensation of urgency or more frequent urination.

3. Sugary and Artificially Sweetened Carbonated Drinks

- Increased Urination in Some Cases: The sugar or artificial sweeteners can also stimulate the bladder, especially in individuals with sensitive bladders or conditions like overactive bladder syndrome.

4. Alcoholic Carbonated Drinks (e.g., Beer, Hard Seltzer)

- Diuretic Effect of Alcohol: Alcohol inhibits the release of vasopressin, a hormone that helps your kidneys retain water, leading to increased urine output.

As you review these tips, remember that it's perfectly normal to have "off" nights. Be gentle with yourself through this transition. If sleep disturbances persist despite your diligent efforts, it may be worth discussing cognitive-behavioral therapy (CBT) for insomnia with healthcare professionals, especially those experienced with menopause. This therapeutic approach has shown promise in helping improve sleep patterns among menopausal women (Drake et al., 2019).

What About the Mood Swings?

Ever find yourself on an emotional roller coaster that rivals the wildest amusement park rides? As you hang on for dear life, remember, it's not all in your head—it's also in your body. Hormonal changes during menopause and perimenopause can lead to mood swings that seem to turn your world upside-down. Honestly, the last time I felt like this, I believe I was smack in the middle of puberty!

Before you decide to run away with the circus, let's look at how these hormonal fluctuations influence your mood—and, more importantly, how you can ride those waves with a little more grace and humor.

First, understanding the science behind mood swings is imperative. Our bodies are finely tuned machines, and hormones are their invisible conductors. Estrogen, progesterone, and even testosterone take turns playing the leading roles, their levels fluctuating as unpredictably as a cat on catnip. When estrogen dips, serotonin levels might follow suit, creating a cascading effect that could result in everything from irritability to anxiety to a crying fit over a sappy TV commercial.

Recognizing these influences validates your feelings and helps reduce that nagging sense of isolation. Just knowing that you're not alone in this can be a relief, like finding out someone else has survived a family holiday dinner without torching the turkey.

What the Man in My Life Needs to Know About My Mood Swings

Ladies and gentlemen, gather around! I'm about to share a little insight into a phenomenon that has baffled men for ages: my mood swings. Picture this: We're enjoying a lovely afternoon, the sun is shining, then suddenly, without warning, I'm in tears over a commercial about puppies. No, I'm not unbalanced; I'm battling the chaos of emotions courtesy of good old menopause!

Share this part with the man in your life!

These swings do not reflect your stability or sanity. Instead, they're the result of your body undergoing significant changes—hormonal adjustments that can feel terrifying and uncomfortable. One minute, you can be cheerful and energetic, ready to conquer the world, and the next, you might need a box of tissues and a cozy blanket.

So, why does this happen? Hormones, hormones, hormones! They're like uninvited guests throwing a rave in your body, and you are just trying to manage the mayhem. A combination of estrogen and progesterone fluctuations can lead to these emotional ups and downs, and while they may not make much sense to him, be assured that they're very real for you.

How Can Your Partner Help?

Now that your guy has a glimpse into your emotional mania, here's how the incredible man in your life can step in and offer support:

- **Be patient:** Sometimes your mood swings may seem irrational. Remember, you are not trying to be difficult; you might need some time and understanding to get through them. Patience goes a long way!

- **Validate feelings:** It can be incredibly reassuring when he acknowledges what you are going through. Phrases such as "I can see that this is tough for you" or "I'm here for you" can make a world of difference.

- **Offer practical help:** Whether it's preparing a cup of tea, suggesting a walk, or taking over chores when you are feeling overwhelmed, his willingness to lend a hand can be comforting and is appreciated.

- **Educate yourself:** Ask him to consider reading up on menopause to better understand what you are experiencing. Knowledge is power, enabling him to respond with empathy rather than confusion (Psst, this is a great book!)

- **Just be there:** Sometimes, the most reassuring thing he can do is to be present. Ask him to try holding your hand during a challenging moment or spending some quiet time with you.

Managing your mood swings during menopause is a process that you don't have to take on alone. Tell him, With your compassion and support, we can make it through this unpredictable phase together, armed with laughter, love, and a better understanding of each other. Let's embrace this adventure, shall we?

Watch Out for Those Triggers

Identifying the specific triggers that intensify your mood swings is the next step toward reclaiming control. Perhaps it's stress, lack of sleep, or the disappearance of your favorite comfy pants (seriously, where do they go?). Some women notice patterns tied to their menstrual cycles, while others might relate their moods to external factors, such as work or family dynamics. Keeping a journal to track these instances might help reveal a common thread, like unraveling a mystery novel's plot twists. Once these triggers have been unveiled, you gain the power to implement changes that can stabilize your moods, turning you from the Mr. Hyde of yesterday into the calm and collected Dr. Jekyll of tomorrow.

Handling Mood Swings with Ease

Now, onto the good stuff—coping strategies! Think of them as your trusty toolbox filled with gadgets ready to tackle any emotional hurricane.

Incorporating mindfulness techniques can help center your thoughts and emotions. Apps designed for meditation and deep-breathing exercises are great places to start, allowing you to transform a moment of turmoil into an oasis of calm. Picture yourself as a leaf floating on a tranquil pond—Zen vibes activated!

Physical activity is another fantastic way to manage mood swings. Exercise releases endorphins, which are basically party planners for your brain and can improve the stability of your mood. Walking your fur baby should bring a smile to your face, or try a dance party in your living room where nobody judges your '90s moves. Staying active isn't just about tightening buns; it's about lifting spirits, too.

Finally, don't underestimate the power of open communication when managing emotional fluctuations. Sharing your feelings with friends, family, or support groups provides community support that reminds you, again, that you're not alone. Imagine being part of a club where everyone gets it, like belonging to a book club where the first rule is to bring wine and empathy.

Incorporating these techniques offers benefits beyond mood regulation and fosters a holistic approach to wellness. Acknowledging the impact of hormonal changes allows you to develop self-compassion.

Unpacking Brain Fog

Menopause brings many changes, and the one that many women find particularly challenging is the infamous "brain fog." You know, that feeling when you walk into a room and forget why you're there or blank on a familiar name mid-conversation? It's a universal experience, but can be particularly pronounced during menopause. For me, it's name recall!

First, let's clarify what brain fog is. Although it's not an official medical term, it aptly describes this specific blend of forgetfulness, confusion, and lack of focus. During menopause, these cognitive changes aren't just imaginary; up to two-thirds of women transitioning through this stage experience them, making acceptance and validation key (Marcin, 2024).

So, what causes this cerebral cloudiness? Several factors might contribute, including hormonal changes and lifestyle influences. As women age, their levels of estrogen—an essential hormone for cognitive function—decline. This decrease can affect memory and mental clarity. Meanwhile, stress frequently intensifies during menopause due to both internal changes and external life pressures. Lifestyle plays a role, too; lack of sleep, poor diet, and minimal exercise can exacerbate those foggy moments. These factors highlight the interconnected nature of cognitive challenges during menopause.

How to Fight Back Against Brain Fog

Now, on to fighting back against brain fog. While it may feel as if your brain's Wi-Fi connection is dropping in and out, there are several strategies to help boost its signal. Using memory aids is a fantastic starting point. For instance, simple tools like lists, calendars, and alarms can turn chaos into order, helping you structure your daily activities and reducing anxiety and forgetfulness. Keeping a diary or planner will also prove beneficial for tracking important information and deadlines.

Promoting brain health through continuous learning is another helpful strategy. Engaging your brain with new challenges stimulates capacity and growth. Let's say you decide learning French is all the rage, or putting together puzzles of kittens, or maybe you fancy mastering a musical instrument? Consider these activities a workout for your brain, strengthening its connections and adapting to new patterns. Learning keeps the mind agile. Voila!

Physical activity cannot be underestimated, either. Regular exercise nourishes the brain with increased blood flow and oxygen, enhancing overall cognitive function (Marcin, 2024). You don't need to train for the Olympics, though! Fit simple activities such as walking or yoga into your daily routines as they offer immense benefits. Committing to consistent exercise can reduce the brain fog's hold on your mind.

Bringing It All Together

The world of menopause can feel like an epic quest filled with mysterious challenges, like hot flashes that appear from nowhere and night sweats that are determined to drench your dreams. In this chapter, we've moved through the landscape of these common symptoms, figuring out how they throw our daily lives into a whirlwind. But, armed with knowledge about hormonal shenanigans and a few practical tips, you're set to tame these fiery and sweaty dragons. From sipping calming herbal teas instead of electrifying coffee to embracing cooling gadgets such as fans and breathable linens, your toolbox is now stocked with ways to turn nighttime disturbances into peaceful slumber.

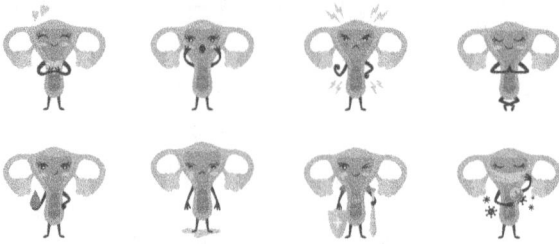

Remember, you're on this trek with countless other women who understand exactly what you're going through. So, welcome self-compassion and resilience; each challenge is a chance for growth and connection. Together, we can laugh, learn a lot, and make this transition as smooth (and cool) as possible.

Chapter Four

The Emotional Rollercoaster (And How to Enjoy the Ride)

T he fluctuating hormones during menopause can make every day feel like you're auditioning for a dramatic role. While mood swings might be an unwanted co-star, they don't have to overshadow the performance. Welcome these emotions as part of a greater script that highlights resilience and personal growth. In doing so, you'll find yourself equipped to handle both the chaos and the calmness that menopause offers.

In this chapter, we'll jump into the nuanced world of the emotional and mental challenges faced during menopause. We'll address the societal expectations that often hush open conversations about vulnerability, creating an environment where keeping silent seems easier than sharing the truth.

We'll also explore how discussing feelings can create a sense of community and understanding among women going through similar experiences, because sometimes, it helps to know you're not the only one fighting off the hot flashes while simultaneously debating if having an ice cream counts as self-care. Through reflective techniques and candid discussions, this chapter will enable you to face menopause with a smile, armed with knowledge, a supportive community, and maybe a stash of chocolate hidden in your sock drawer for those tough days!

Managing Emotional Chaos: It's Normal

Embracing the whirlwind of emotions during menopause is not just normal; it's empowering. Understanding and managing these changes is key to taking control of your experience. Society has long imposed the expectation for women to maintain an ever-cool demeanor. Be it at home, work, or elsewhere, the pressure to stay composed (even while dripping sweat) often discourages the expression of emotions, leading many to silently endure their struggles.

While silent endurance can seem like strength, openly discussing your feelings may promote a more profound understanding and acceptance of the emotional chaos that comes with menopause. When we share our experiences, we create a space where other women can come forward and talk about theirs, too. Acknowledging these feelings openly can shift perceptions and reduce the stigma associated with showing vulnerability during menopause.

Let's face it—menopause isn't all about crying or laughing because your keys are missing. It challenges your psyche. The mental gymnastics you perform daily, from ecstatic to inexplicably melancholic, are not imagined. They're deeply rooted in hormonal changes, societal pressures, and personal expectations. By validating and vocalizing what you're experiencing, you improve your mental health, turning acknowledgment into empowerment.

Untangling Social Stigma

For years, conversations around menopause have been wrapped in euphemisms, whispers, or even jokes. But while humor can bring discussions into the light, it often trivializes genuine experiences. All older women would be rich if they had a dollar for every time a family member asked, "Are you moody today because of 'the menopause'?" Recognizing menopause as a natural life transition rather than a punchline can elevate our discourse to one of respect and empathy. Women who speak candidly about their challenges help dismantle the silence shrouding this topic and contribute to creating supportive networks.

Now, let's unravel how societal expectations play a role. Have you ever felt the need to soldier through your day despite feeling off-kilter emotionally? Many cultures perpetuate the idea that women must appear unshakable and relegate authentic emotions to the background. This pressure can lead to emotional suppression and increased stress levels, further complicating the menopausal transition. For instance, the expectation to always be "put together" can make it difficult to express when you're feeling overwhelmed by menopausal symptoms.

Imagine a world where expressing emotions doesn't equate to weakness, but is a testament to your resilience, honesty, and openness. Engaging in open dialogue with friends, family, or support groups can break down barriers, illuminating the shared human experience of menopause and creating collective strength. When we open up about our feelings, we support our own healing and enable others to do the same.

Impact of Relationships on Emotions: How Menopause Affects Personal Connections

Relationships play a significant role in shaping our emotions. During menopause, that connection can be influenced in substantial ways. As our hormone levels fluctuate, so do our moods and feelings, which can create ripples in our relationships with partners, family, and friends. For instance, sudden mood swings can lead to misunderstandings or tension with your partner. However, open and honest communication can pave the way for understanding, support, and strengthened bonds.

Menopause isn't a solitary journey; it affects those around us, too. Partners may feel confused or helpless when faced with sudden mood changes, leading to tension and a lack of connection. However, it's essential to remember that this shared experience can bring couples closer together if addressed openly. Also, knowing that others are going through similar experiences can provide a sense of connection and support.

Building Strong Support Systems

When both partners feel equipped to discuss feelings, fears, and experiences, they can find comfort in knowing they're supported. Building these open lines of communication can help both people understand each other better, creating a sense of partnership and unity during challenging times.

Having these conversations during menopause can strengthen relationships and create mutual understanding—for instance, realizing both partners now need to bring an extra fan into the bedroom. Partners can support each other, listen to each other's concerns, and work together to find solutions, whether attending a doctor's appointment or engaging in self-care practices such as synchronized ice cream eating during hot flashes!

Questions to Encourage Open Discussion

To start the conversation about menopause and emotional well-being with your partner, consider these questions:

- What feelings or concerns do you have about menopause, and how does it impact our relationship?

- Have there been specific moments or situations where you felt unsure about how to support me?

- How do you feel about discussing menopause and its challenges together?

- What are some ways we can stay connected and supportive during this time?

- How can I help you better understand what I'm going through?

- Is there anything you could do to help me during this time?

- What activities can we engage in together to strengthen our relationship?

- How can we establish a routine where we regularly discuss our feelings, needs, and concerns?

Encouraging your partner to express their feelings is just as important! By asking them how they feel and what they need, you create a reciprocal dynamic where you both feel heard and supported.

Menopause can present unique challenges to relationships, but it also serves as an opportunity for growth, empathy, and understanding. Remember, love and communication are the keys to handling life's changes together. Open and honest communication can pave the way for understanding, support, and strengthened bonds, reassuring both partners that they are understood and supported.

Ellen's Menopause Moment: From Punchline to Powerhouse

Ellen had always been the glue that held her household together. She was the finder of lost shoes, the maker of lasagna, and the woman who knew exactly when her husband was sick versus when he just had a man cold. Lately, however, she has felt more like the frayed edges of that glue, held together by sheer willpower and maybe a second glass of wine on a Tuesday.

Menopause had come in like a wrecking ball. She couldn't sleep; her body felt as if it were hosting an internal furnace, and her emotions were running wild. One minute, she yelled at the dog for breathing too loudly; the next, she was sobbing over a commercial for paper towels. But what truly pushed her over the edge wasn't the hot flashes or the brain fog—it was the *jokes*.

Her husband, Mike, and their 15-year-old son, Jason, had become a comedy duo with Ellen as their main material.

"Mom lost her glasses again," Jason would quip, imitating her frantic searching.

"Honey, are you hot again? It's practically the Arctic in here," Mike would add, adjusting the thermostat as if he were auditioning for *The Price Is Right*.

And they exchanged "the look" when Ellen burst into tears mid-dinner over a particularly soggy taco shell. That "What do we do with her?" look that made her want to throw the taco shell at them both.

One night, as Mike adjusted the thermostat for the third time in an hour, Ellen snapped. "Step away from the thermostat!" she shouted. Silence filled the room. Even the dog stopped chewing his bone.

She stood there; her face flushed (from rage or a hot flash; it was hard to tell) and realized: enough was enough.

The next day, Ellen called a family meeting. Jason showed up with his headphones still dangling from his ears while Mike shuffled in, holding a cup of coffee like a shield. They sat down at the kitchen table—the very table where Ellen had solved Jason's childhood crises, her and Mike's work dilemmas, and, yes, both of their digestive issues.

She took a deep breath. "We need to talk. And I need you both to listen."

Mike raised an eyebrow, and Jason gave her his patented teenager slouch, but she pressed on.

"I love you both. But I can't keep being the punchline to your menopause jokes. I know you think it's harmless, but it's not. You don't understand what I'm going through—physically, emotionally, mentally. And frankly, I don't blame you. I didn't understand teething or potty training or your hormones during puberty either, Jason. But you know what I did? I educated myself. For you. And Mike," she added, fixing her husband with a steely glare, "when you were struggling with your ... ahem, constipation issues last year, who read up on every possible solution?"

Mike shifted uncomfortably. "You did," he mumbled.

"Exactly. Now it's your turn to help. I need support and love—not jokes. I've printed out some information for you." She slid a stack of papers across the table. "Read it. Learn the science. Understand what I'm going through."

Jason looked horrified. "Is this mandatory?"

"Of course," Ellen said sternly. "Because the next time one of you cracks a joke about me being hot or losing my glasses, I'm handing over a comprehensive guide to my symptoms. And trust me, it's a minimum of 500 pages."

To Ellen's surprise, they took her seriously. Over the next week, Jason actually read the articles she'd printed, occasionally muttering things like, "Wow, I didn't know that could happen." Mike watched a few videos she'd recommended, even pausing the football to ask her questions about HRT.

And the jokes? They stopped.

Instead, Ellen's men began supporting her in small but meaningful ways. Jason offered to help find her glasses without making a sarcastic comment. Mike gave his wife complete control of the thermostat and bought a few extra sweaters for himself. They even began asking if they could help and how she was doing.

One night, Ellen accidentally set off the smoke alarm while cooking dinner, and for the first time in weeks, everyone laughed—including Ellen. "Well, at least I didn't lose my glasses this time!" she joked. They all burst into laughter, but it felt different. It wasn't laughter *at* her—it was laughter *with* her.

In the months that followed, Ellen felt the shift in her household. Her husband and son didn't just understand her better—they also respected her more. Menopause was no longer something to joke about; it was just a part of their lives, like Jason's endless quest to grow facial hair or Mike's obsessive lawn-mowing schedule.

And Ellen? She felt lighter, more liberated, and deeply grateful. Sometimes, all it takes is a little education, a lot of honesty, and a well-timed family meeting to remind everyone that love and support matter.

Addressing Depression and Anxiety: Breaking the Silence

During menopause, many women find themselves grappling with unexpected mental health challenges. You're going through a life change, and while everyone around you seems to be focusing on the physical symptoms, it may be the emotional turbulence that knocks you flying. Research shows that a large percentage of women experience depression and anxiety during menopause, and in one study, anxiety symptoms increased from 3.1% before menopause to 7.0% during and 7.4% after menopause. Knowing these statistics can be the first step in understanding that these feelings aren't uncommon.

Symptoms and Breaking the Stigma

According to a 2024 study from the North American Menopause Society, nearly 60% of women report mood disturbances during perimenopause, but fewer than 25% seek treatment. Recognizing that menopause can impact your mental health is important for managing it effectively. Let's break down the symptoms that differentiate a lousy day from something more concerning. Typical life stressors might cause fleeting moments of anxiety or low mood. However, it's time to notice if these emotions linger and interfere with your daily life. Symptoms such as persistent sadness, irritability, difficulty concentrating, and overwhelming fatigue aren't just par for the menopausal course; they can signal deeper struggles.

Acknowledging these issues leads us to the next important point: smashing the stigma surrounding mental health during menopause. For too long, talking about mental health has been taboo, shared behind closed doors rather than discussed openly at the breakfast table. Now, it's time to change that story. By sharing our experiences and listening to the stories of others, we diminish the stigma and create a culture of support and understanding. Whether it's a chat over coffee or joining an online community, speaking up can be surprisingly supportive.

Cognitive behavioral therapy (CBT) and SSRIs/SNRIs can reduce mood symptoms during menopause. The menu is vast: CBT, HRT, counseling, and mindfulness exercises are just a few available routes. Treatments should be tailored to fit your needs, much like choosing the perfect pair of shoes—comfortable, supportive, and stylish. Some women benefit from medication, while others find comfort in lifestyle changes, such as regular exercise and a balanced diet. Think of it as a holistic tune-up for both mind and body. Maybe it's yoga one day and a brisk walk in the park the next. Every little bit helps.

Now, when it comes to seeking help, don't delay. Mental health challenges during menopause aren't figments of your imagination; they're genuine and deserve attention. Your primary care doctor can be a starting point, offering guidance and support tailored to your situation. By reaching out, you can take control of your mental well-being and advocate for the care you deserve.

The Mood-Body Connection: New Frontiers in Mental Wellness

Let's talk about something that's changing how we think about mood during menopause: the realization that your emotional well-being isn't just about your hormones or your thoughts. It involves your entire body system, from your genes to your gut bacteria. Welcome to the world of precision psychiatry and the gut-brain axis.

Precision Psychiatry: Finding Your Medication Match

Remember playing pin the tail on the donkey as a kid? That's pretty much how we've been prescribing psychiatric medications for decades. Your doctor guesses which antidepressant might work, you try it for 6-8 weeks, and if it doesn't work (or causes unbearable side effects), you try another one. Rinse and repeat until something sticks.

For women dealing with menopause-related depression or anxiety, this trial-and-error approach is particularly frustrating. You're already struggling with mood swings, brain fog, and hot flashes. The last thing you need is to waste six months on medications that don't work or make you feel worse.

Enter precision psychiatry: using genetic testing to predict which psychiatric medications will work best for you before you even take the first pill.

Pharmacogenetic Testing: Your Medication Roadmap

Pharmacogenetic testing analyzes genes that control how your body processes medications. It's like having a user manual for your brain's medication receptors.

The CYP450 Genes: These genes determine how fast or slow your liver breaks down medications. They come in several varieties (CYP2D6, CYP2C19, CYP3A4, and others), and your variants dramatically affect medication response.

Poor metabolizers: You break down medications very slowly. Standard doses might build up to toxic levels, causing severe side effects. You need lower doses or different medications entirely.

Ultrarapid metabolizers: You break down medications so fast that they barely have time to work. Standard doses might feel like you're taking nothing at all. You need higher doses or medications that aren't affected by these pathways.

What this means for menopause mood issues: If you're prescribed an SSRI (selective serotonin reuptake inhibitor) like sertraline or escitalopram for depression or hot flashes, your CYP2C19 status predicts how you'll respond. Ultrarapid metabolizers often get zero benefit from standard doses. Poor metabolizers might experience terrible nausea, fatigue, or other side effects at doses that others tolerate fine.

A simple cheek swab can tell you all this before you waste months feeling miserable.

The Serotonin Receptor and Transporter Genes: We mentioned the serotonin transporter gene (5-HTTLPR) earlier. But there are also genes for serotonin receptors (HTR1A, HTR2A, HTR2C) that affect how well SSRIs and SNRIs (serotonin-norepinephrine reuptake inhibitors) work for you.

Women with certain **HTR2A variant**s, for example, are much more likely to experience weight gain on SSRIs. If you know this ahead of time, your doctor might choose a different medication class or add strategies to prevent weight gain.

The MTHFR Gene: This gene affects how your body processes folate (vitamin B9), which is essential for making neurotransmitters like serotonin and dopamine. About 40% of people have MTHFR variants that reduce enzyme function.

If you have MTHFR variants and you're depressed during menopause, you might need L-methylfolate supplementation (the active form of folate your body can actually use) in addition to antidepressants. Some women with treatment-resistant depression finally improve when this is addressed.

The COMT Gene (Revisited): Remember the "warrior vs. worrier" gene from Chapter Two? Your COMT status also predicts medication response. "Warriors" (Val/Val) might respond better to stimulating antidepressants like bupropion. "Worriers" (Met/Met) might do better with calming medications like SSRIs.

Real-World Precision Psychiatry

Here's what this looks like in practice:

Traditional approach: "Let's try Zoloft. If it doesn't work in 6-8 weeks, we'll try Prozac. If that doesn't work, we'll try Wellbutrin ..."

Precision psychiatry approach: "Your genetic test shows you're a CYP2D6 poor metabolizer and a CYP2C19 intermediate metabolizer. You also have the MTHFR C677T variant.

Armed with this information, your plan might look like this: avoid paroxetine (Paxil) and fluoxetine (Prozac) as you'll metabolize them too slowly. Sertraline (Zoloft) should work, but start at half the usual dose, then add L-methylfolate 15 mg daily to support neurotransmitter production. Your serotonin transporter genotype suggests that you'll respond well to SSRIs, and your doctor would recheck in 2-3 weeks instead of waiting 8 weeks.

No more Russian roulette with medications. No more suffering through side effects from drugs that were never going to work for your unique biology.

Current Availability

Several companies now offer pharmacogenetic testing panels:

- **GeneSight** (most widely known, covered by many insurers)

- **Genomind**

- **Myriad Neuroscience**

- **Tempus**

These tests typically cost $300-$2,000, though insurance coverage is improving. Medicare covers some testing in certain circumstances. The test is done once in your lifetime since your genes don't change.

The Gut-Brain Axis: Your Second Brain

Now let's talk about something that sounds like pseudoscience until you dig into the research: your gut bacteria significantly affect your mood during menopause.

Your digestive system contains about 100 trillion bacteria (your microbiome), and these little critters are in constant communication with your brain via the vagus nerve, immune system, and production of neurotransmitters.

Here's the wild part: about 90% of your body's serotonin is produced in your gut, not your brain. Your gut bacteria play a huge role in this production. They also produce GABA (your brain's calming neurotransmitter), dopamine, and other mood-regulating chemicals.

How Menopause Disrupts Your Gut

Estrogen doesn't just affect your reproductive organs and brain. It also shapes your gut microbiome. When estrogen drops during menopause, your gut bacteria composition changes dramatically.

What happens:

- Beneficial bacteria (like Lactobacillus) decline

- Inflammatory bacteria increase

- Gut barrier integrity weakens ("leaky gut")

- Production of mood-supporting metabolites decreases

- Inflammation increases throughout your body, including your brain

This helps explain why some women develop depression, anxiety, or brain fog during menopause even when their psychological stressors haven't changed. Their gut ecosystem has been disrupted.

Gut-Brain Interventions for Mood Stabilization

The exciting news: you can modify your gut microbiome to support better mood during menopause. Here's how:

1. Psychobiotics: Probiotics That Target Mental Health

Not all probiotics are created equal. Certain strains specifically improve mood and anxiety:

Lactobacillus helveticus R0052 and Bifidobacterium longum R0175: This combination has been studied specifically for stress and anxiety. In clinical trials, people taking this combo for 30 days showed significant reductions in anxiety and depression scores.

Lactobacillus rhamnosus: Studies show this strain reduces anxiety-like behavior and lowers stress hormone levels. It works by affecting GABA receptors in the brain.

Bifidobacterium infantis: Particularly good for depression. In one study, this strain was as effective as the antidepressant citalopram at reducing depressive symptoms.

What to look for: Multi-strain probiotics containing at least 10-20 billion CFUs (colony-forming units) of the strains listed above. Take them consistently for at least 8-12 weeks to see mood effects.

2. Prebiotics: Feeding Your Good Bacteria

Prebiotics are food for your beneficial bacteria. They're non-digestible fibers that ferment in your gut and produce helpful metabolites.

Key prebiotics for mood:

- Inulin (found in chicory root, garlic, onions, asparagus)

- Fructooligosaccharides/FOS (found in bananas, wheat, onions)

- Galactooligosaccharides/GOS (found in legumes, certain supplements)

Studies show that prebiotic supplementation reduces cortisol (stress hormone) levels and improves emotional processing. One study found that people taking prebiotics showed reduced attention to negative information, suggesting improved mood regulation.

Practical approach: Eat 25-35 grams of fiber daily, emphasizing prebiotic-rich foods. Alternatively, supplement with 5-10 grams of prebiotic powder daily (start low to avoid gas and bloating).

3. Polyphenols: Plant Compounds that Support Mood

Polyphenols are compounds found in colorful fruits, vegetables, tea, coffee, and dark chocolate. They act as food for beneficial bacteria and have direct anti-inflammatory and neuroprotective effects.

Top polyphenol sources for mood:

- Green tea (L-theanine plus polyphenols = anxiety reduction)

- Blueberries (anthocyanins improve cognitive function)

- Dark chocolate 70%+ cacao (improves mood and supports beneficial bacteria)

- Extra virgin olive oil (oleuropein supports brain health)

- Coffee (yes, coffee! Moderate consumption is associated with reduced depression risk)

The mechanism: Polyphenols are metabolized by gut bacteria into bioactive compounds that cross the blood-brain barrier and reduce brain inflammation. They also increase BDNF (brain-derived neurotrophic factor), which supports brain cell growth and resilience.

4. Fermented Foods: Traditional Wisdom Meets Modern Science

Fermented foods contain live bacteria and bioactive metabolites that support gut and brain health.

Best fermented foods for mood:

- Kefir (dairy or water-based)

- Sauerkraut (unpasteurized)

- Kimchi

- Plain yogurt with live cultures

- Kombucha (watch the sugar content)

- Miso

How much: Aim for 1-2 servings daily. Even small amounts provide billions of beneficial bacteria.

5. The Anti-Inflammatory Diet for Mood

Chronic inflammation is a major driver of depression and anxiety. Your gut bacteria play a huge role in either promoting or reducing inflammation.

Foods that reduce inflammation and support mood:

- Fatty fish (salmon, sardines, mackerel) - omega-3s are powerful anti-inflammatories

- Leafy greens - rich in folate for neurotransmitter production

- Nuts and seeds - especially walnuts for omega-3s

- Berries - antioxidants that reduce brain inflammation

- Turmeric - curcumin crosses the blood-brain barrier and reduces inflammation

Foods that increase inflammation and worsen mood:

- Processed foods with artificial additives

- High-sugar foods (feed inflammatory bacteria)

- Trans fats (directly damage brain cell membranes)

- Excessive alcohol (disrupts gut barrier, reduces beneficial bacteria)

- Artificial sweeteners (disrupt gut bacteria balance)

6. Omega-3 Fatty Acids: The Gut-Brain Bridge

Omega-3s deserve special mention because they work on multiple levels:

- Reduce gut inflammation

- Support beneficial bacteria growth

- Directly reduce brain inflammation

- Are building blocks for brain cell membranes

- Help produce mood-regulating neurotransmitters

Clinical trials show that omega-3 supplementation (particularly EPA) reduces depression symptoms, with effects comparable to some antidepressants.

Dosage for mood: 1,000-2,000mg of combined EPA+DHA daily, with at least 60% as EPA. Use high-quality fish oil or algae-based omega-3s for vegetarians.

Integrating Gut-Brain and Precision Psychiatry Approaches

The most powerful approach combines these strategies:

> **Example Protocol for Menopausal Depression:**
> **Week 1-2:**
> Get pharmacogenetic testing done
> Start probiotic with Lactobacillus helveticus and Bifidobacterium longum
> Add 2,000 mg omega-3 daily
> Eliminate inflammatory foods, add fermented foods
> **Week 3-4:**
> Receive genetic results
> Start medication based on genetic guidance (or continue medication adjustment)
> Add prebiotic fiber supplement
> Increase polyphenol-rich foods
> **Week 6-8:**
> Reassess mood and symptoms
> Adjust medications if needed (but give gut interventions time to work)
> Consider adding L-methylfolate if MTHFR variants present
> Continue gut-supportive diet
> **Week 12:**
> Evaluate overall response
> Fine-tune approach based on what's working
> Consider adding mind-body practices (meditation, yoga) for additional support

The Hormone-Gut-Mood Triangle

Here's where it gets really interesting: HRT, gut health, and mood are interconnected.

Some women start HRT, and their mood improves not just because of direct brain effects, but also because estrogen helps restore beneficial gut bacteria. Other women improve their gut health and find they need less HRT or lower doses because their overall inflammation decreases.

The ideal approach addresses all three:

- **Hormones** (HRT if appropriate)

- **Gut health** (probiotics, prebiotics, diet)

- **Brain chemistry** (medications if needed, targeted to your genetics)

Testing Your Gut Microbiome

COMPANY	WHAT IT MEASURES	WHAT YOU RECEIVE	~COST	NOTES
Viome	Levels of beneficial and inflammatory bacteria, overall microbiome diversity	Personalized food and supplement recommendations based on your gut profile	$149 - $399	Focuses on linking gut health to energy, metabolism, and mood
Thorne	Bacterial balance and gut inflammation markers	Detailed gut health report and dietary guidance	$199 - $299	Integrates with Thorne's supplement ecosystem for customized plans
Ombre	Diversity of your microbiome and ratios of beneficial vs. harmful strains	Personalized probiotic and food recommendations	$99 - $129	User-friendly app for tracking progress and symptom changes
Tiny Health	Beneficial and inflammatory bacteria, diversity metrics	Family-focused insights with food and supplement suggestions	$150 - $350	Designed for women, infants, and families—tracks gut health over time

NOTE: While these tests aren't yet considered standard medical care, they can offer helpful insights—especially if you're experiencing persistent digestive or mood issues that haven't improved with conventional treatment.

What Your Doctor Might Not Know

Here's the truth: most doctors didn't learn about pharmacogenetics or the gut-brain axis in medical school. This is cutting-edge stuff, and it takes time for new research to filter into clinical practice.

If your doctor isn't familiar with these approaches, you're not stuck. You can ask for a referral to a psychiatrist who specializes in pharmacogenomics, consult with a functional medicine practitioner, or work with an integrative psychiatrist.

Some women find that combining conventional care (from their regular doctor) with functional medicine consultation (for gut-brain interventions) works well.

The Bottom Line on Mood and Menopause

Depression and anxiety during menopause aren't character flaws or just "part of getting older." They're biological phenomena with biological solutions.

The future of treating mood issues during menopause involves:

Precision psychiatry: Right medication, right dose, first time

Gut-brain interventions: Supporting the microbiome to support your mood

Personalized approaches: Based on your genetics, microbiome, hormones, and life circumstances

You don't have to accept suffering as inevitable, and you don't have to play medication roulette for months on end. The tools exist now to personalize your treatment and dramatically improve your chances of feeling better faster.

Your mood matters. Your quality of life matters. You deserve treatment that actually works for your unique biology.

Cognitive Changes and Mental Clarity

While menopause can be a time of liberation and self-discovery, let's not forget the cognitive changes accompanying the ride (uninvited, some might say).

First up on our parade? Hormonal changes. These relentless little gremlins have quite the talent for shaking things up, particularly estrogen. Estrogen has its hands all over your brain's cognitive functions, including memory and focus. So, it's like the director suddenly went missing from your brain's blockbuster movie set, leaving you with memory lapses, misplaced keys, and blank moments during conversations.

There are several strategies you can use to harness your inner brilliance and keep those cognitive cogs turning smoothly. To start, you can dive into the world of brain exercises. Think of them as gym workouts for your noggin. Engaging in puzzles, solving crosswords, or even picking up a musical instrument can sharpen your mind and improve your memory (*Navigating Memory Changes in Menopause*, 2024). And if you've ever wanted to learn a new language, now's the time. Say goodbye to mundane activities and accept your inner puzzle master.

Next, let's welcome mindfulness. Mindfulness can come from simply being present in the moment. Try focusing on the sensation of brushing your teeth or savoring the aroma of your morning coffee. Regular meditation can also improve your concentration, aligning your thoughts like a chorus singing in perfect harmony.

Here are three simple mindfulness exercises that you can practice anytime to reduce stress and increase awareness:

1. 5-4-3-2-1 Grounding Exercise

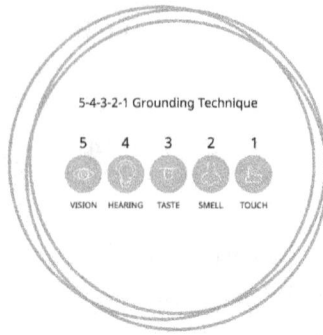

5-4-3-2-1 Grounding Technique

5	4	3	2	1
VISION	HEARING	TASTE	SMELL	TOUCH

This exercise uses your senses to bring you into the present moment:

- Step 1: Take a deep breath.

- Step 2: Identify 5 things you can see around you.

- Step 3: Identify 4 things you can touch (e.g., the texture of your clothes or a nearby object).

- Step 4: Identify 3 things you can hear, focusing on sounds in your environment.

- Step 5: Identify 2 things you can smell (or imagine favorite smells if none are present).

- Step 6: Identify 1 thing you can taste, or focus on the taste in your mouth.

- How It Helps: This exercise engages your senses to reduce anxiety and bring focus to the present.

2. Box Breathing (4-4-4-4 Breathing)

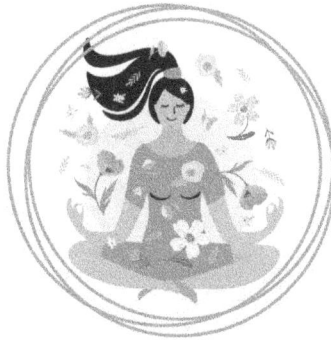

A simple breathing technique that promotes calmness:

- Step 1: Inhale slowly through your nose for a count of 4.

- Step 2: Hold your breath for 4 seconds.

- Step 3: Exhale slowly through your mouth for 4 seconds.

- Step 4: Hold your breath again for 4 seconds.

- Step 5: Repeat for 1-2 minutes.

- How It Helps: Box breathing activates the parasympathetic nervous system, helping to reduce stress and enhance focus.

3. Body Scan Meditation

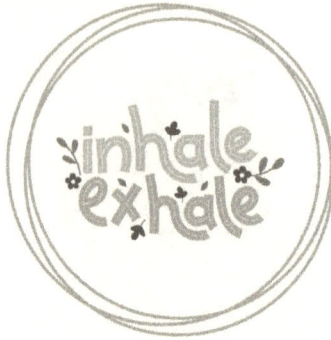

A quick way to connect with your body and release tension:

- Step 1: Sit or lie down comfortably and close your eyes.

- Step 2: Take a few deep breaths to relax.

- Step 3: Slowly bring your attention to your feet, noticing any sensations.

- Step 4: Gradually move your attention up through your legs, hips, abdomen, chest, arms, neck, and head.

- Step 5: If you notice any tension, breathe into that area and imagine it releasing with each exhale.

- How It Helps: A body scan increases awareness of physical sensations and helps reduce stress by promoting relaxation.

Now, we'll turn to the delicious topic of nutrition. Your food isn't just fuel; it's also brain magic. Omega-3 fatty acids are in the spotlight here, playing the hero role by supporting brain health. Indulge in salmon, flaxseeds, and walnuts to treat your gray matter to an omega-3 feast. Antioxidant-rich foods like berries and leafy greens join the cast, ready to battle oxidative stress and protect those precious brain cells. A diet rich in these nutrients can lead to sharper cognition and a happier spirit.

Creating a cognitive-friendly environment is another splendid act in our play. The goal? Making organization your best friend. Keep your surroundings neat and tidy. Label things if needed and banish clutter to allow your brain to breathe freely. Let there be light—natural light, that is! Open those curtains wide during the day. The natural light will nudge you to feel more awake and alert, making cloudy thoughts fade away like mist at sunrise.

Bringing It All Together

The emotional and mental landscape of menopause can be a wild and unpredictable ride, complete with ups, downs, and sideways loops. Throughout this chapter, we've walked through the swirling storm of feelings accompanying menopause and welcomed the chaos instead of pushing it aside. By acknowledging these emotions rather than suppressing them, you can build a healthier mindset where feeling low on some days is as acceptable as celebrating joyful moments on others. Remember, you're not alone; connecting with others can change perceived struggles into shared experiences, creating a beautiful blend of mutual understanding and empathy.

Menopause is an opportunity for growth, learning, and unearthing strengths within yourself that you might have forgotten existed. You can empower yourself and those around you with candid conversations and a dash of reflection. Cherish the ride of emotions as part of the journey, knowing they're carving out a path toward resilience and authenticity during this phase of life.

Chapter Five

HRT Demystified: Your Hormone Cheat Sheet

Hormone replacement therapy (HRT), often shrouded in mystery and skepticism, is an elusive elixir many are curious about but aren't exactly sure how it fits into their lives. This chapter unfolds the story behind HRT, examining its potential to change the menopausal path from an uphill battle to a gentle stroll. We start by lifting the veil of confusion surrounding HRT, presenting it as friend and foe, depending on the narrative you choose to follow. It's like exploring a new city: some streets lead to delightful views, while others require caution signs along the way.

In our exploration, we'll unravel the various benefits that make HRT appealing to many women searching for relief from disruptive symptoms. However, we won't stop at just the good news. The conversation takes a balanced turn, investigating the risks attached to this medical approach as well; think of it as a seesaw, where understanding ensures neither side tips too far. By the end, a trusty guidebook will equip you with the knowledge to empower your decision-making, much like choosing your next adventure.

Understanding HRT

HRT, often perceived as a magic wand for those navigating the choppy waters of menopause, offers a significant upgrade to your body's functioning. It's like downloading a software update that smoothens out the rough patches, especially when dealing with those pesky hot flashes and mood swings. More than just feeling better, HRT is about reclaiming life from the grips of fluctuating hormones.

How HRT Works

Let's dive into how HRT pulls off this magic trick. We've discussed how hormones such as estrogen and progesterone start playing hide-and-seek during menopause, disappearing from their usual hangouts. This is where HRT steps in with its superhero cape, replenishing these essential hormones to bring some balance back to your body. For many, this means bidding farewell to the overbearing heat waves and emotional roller coasters that can leave you frazzled. By tackling these symptoms head-on, HRT can change menopause from a dreaded era into a manageable phase of life.

Now, nothing in life is one-size-fits-all, and HRT is no exception. It's like going to an ice cream shop offering an array of flavors—you've got estrogen-only, combination therapies involving estrogen and progesterone, and even bioidentical hormones made to mimic the body's natural form of estrogen more closely. Each type has its unique formula and purpose, ensuring a perfect scoop (or dose) tailored just for you. Your path with HRT becomes as customized as picking the right ingredients for a recipe and making sure it suits your needs perfectly.

Types of HRT

Moving on to delivery options, consider them like vehicles for getting these hormones to their destination. Whether it's a pill you swallow, a patch stuck on your arm like a fashion statement, or a gel you rub onto your skin as part of your morning routine, each method offers a level of flexibility. You're no longer constrained by limited options; you can choose a treatment plan that fits seamlessly into your lifestyle. It's all about finding what works best for you—kind of like choosing between riding a bike or driving a car, which gets you to work on time without the stress of traffic jams.

At the heart of HRT's effectiveness lies its individualized nature—a concept worth embracing wholeheartedly. Gone are the days of generic treatments; today's HRT landscape is all about personalization. This approach acknowledges that your experiences, health history, and preferences are as unique as your fingerprint, allowing for informed discussions with healthcare providers. When you engage in these candid conversations, you're not just talking about medications; you're also paving a path toward a more comfortable and empowered menopausal experience, making you feel valued and understood.

Educated Discussions with Your Healthcare Provider

In conversation with your healthcare provider, you'll explore the nuances of HRT, dissecting factors such as dosage, forms, and durations. Understanding whether you're a candidate for estrogen-only therapy or if a combination is necessary is a little like selecting a tailor-made outfit. This detailed dialogue will guarantee that your treatment aligns with your health goals while keeping potential risks at bay.

Despite its benefits, you shouldn't take the decision to start HRT lightly. Rather, it's a well-calibrated dance between advantages and risks, each weighed carefully against the other. This may involve reconciling the promise of symptom relief with awareness of the possible side effects, thereby motivating you to delve deeper into your individual considerations. Such deliberations emphasize why personalized care remains vital, because what works fantastically for one person might not work as well for another.

Analyzing the Risks and Benefits of HRT

HRT may offer a smoother track during menopause. As we've seen, many women experience night sweats, hot flashes, and other symptoms that disrupt their lives, a bit like having their own personal sauna that shows up uninvited. For these symptoms, HRT can be beneficial, offering a ray of hope and allowing you to reclaim those hours of sleep or go through your day without feeling as if you're in a constant furnace. The relief provided by HRT is akin to finding the magic ingredient for your perfect cup of coffee in the morning—it makes everything else seem more manageable.

Risks of HRT

Like any potent potion, HRT comes with a few caveats. Our bodies are wonderfully unique, and there's no one-size-fits-all approach. Current guidelines from organizations like The Menopause Society and The American College of Obstetricians and Gynecologists (ACOG) emphasize that HRT should be tailored to each individual's needs, considering age, time since menopause, symptom severity, and personal health history.

The potential health risks associated with HRT, such as an increased chance of breast cancer and blood clots, may sound ominous. The

Women's Health Initiative (WHI) study, along with more recent research, has found that:

- Combined HRT (estrogen + progestin) is associated with a slightly increased risk of breast cancer, particularly with long-term use (over 5 years).

- Estrogen-only HRT, typically prescribed for women who have had a hysterectomy, does not appear to increase breast cancer risk and may reduce it slightly.

- Blood Clots: All forms of systemic HRT can increase the risk of venous thromboembolism (VTE), especially with oral formulations. However, transdermal patches and gels may present a lower risk.

Next, you must have a detailed understanding of your personal and family medical history and assess such regarding the benefit-risk ratio of HRT.

Risk factors like a history of breast cancer, heart disease, stroke, or blood clots significantly influence the safety and suitability of HRT for each individual. Consulting with healthcare providers familiar with your history is imperative to ensure you're getting relief and doing so safely. Experts recommend regular monitoring and re-evaluation of HRT, especially as health status or symptoms change. While HRT can be beneficial, it's not something you set and forget, like a Crock-Pot cooking dinner. Regular monitoring and re-evaluation with your healthcare provider are essential components in effectively managing ongoing risks. Think of it as scheduling regular maintenance checks for your beloved car; you wouldn't want to skip them and end up with a surprise breakdown on the highway.

On the path to making an informed decision about whether HRT is right for you, the best approach involves weighing personal factors and seeking advice from multiple professionals. It's the same as preparing for any significant life event—gathering different perspectives leads to a well-rounded choice. Picture yourself assembling a dream team of experts who bring diverse insights to help shape your story. From your primary care doctor and gynecologist to perhaps even an endocrinologist, each piece of advice contributes to a comprehensive understanding, ensuring you're confident in your decision.

When considering HRT, you must ask all the questions swirling around in your head. Approach it as if you're interviewing where you're the star journalist, probing for answers that help uncover the truth about what will work best for you. Your healthcare provider should support this exploration process, be ready to guide you through the pros and cons, and ensure you're equipped with all the information before deciding.

Remember, hormone therapy isn't a lifelong commitment unless you decide it is. It can act as a bridge through particularly challenging periods, offering support and relief when needed most. Just like wearing layers in fickle weather, you have the flexibility to adapt and change based on how you're feeling and what's happening in your life.

The Cutting Edge: What Your Doctor Might Not Know Yet

Let's talk about the cool stuff happening in menopause treatment right now. While your mom might have had two choices (suffer silently or take the same HRT pill as everyone else), you're living in a time when menopause medicine is getting a serious upgrade. Think of it like going from flip phones to smartphones. The basics still work, but wow, the new features are impressive.

Menopause Biomarkers: Your Body's Personal Report Card

Remember when diagnosing menopause was basically your doctor shrugging and saying, "Well, you haven't had a period in 12 months, so... menopause"? Those days are fading fast. Now we have biomarkers, which are basically your body's way of texting you updates about what's happening with your hormones.

What Are These Biomarkers Anyway?

Biomarkers are measurable indicators in your blood that tell the story of your hormonal journey. The main players include:

Follicle-Stimulating Hormone (FSH): Think of FSH as your ovaries' increasingly desperate wake-up call. As you approach menopause, your brain cranks up FSH production, trying to get your ovaries to respond. It's like when you keep turning up the volume on your phone alarm, but your body just hits snooze. High FSH levels (typically over 25-30 mIU/mL) suggest you're in perimenopause or beyond.

Estradiol (E2): This is the main estrogen your ovaries produce during your reproductive years. As menopause approaches, estradiol levels drop. Low estradiol (typically under 30 pg/mL) combined with high FSH is a pretty clear sign that menopause has arrived at your doorstep, probably without calling first.

Anti-Müllerian Hormone (AMH): This one's newer to the menopause conversation. AMH levels reflect your ovarian reserve, basically telling you how many eggs you have left in the carton. As you approach menopause, AMH drops to nearly undetectable levels. It's like watching your phone battery go from 15% to 1%.

Why Should You Care About These Numbers?

Here's the thing: knowing your biomarker levels isn't just about confirming you're in menopause. It's about predicting what's coming and personalizing your treatment. Some women with specific biomarker patterns experience more severe symptoms. Others might have higher risks for bone loss or cardiovascular issues. When your doctor knows your numbers, they can create a treatment plan that's actually designed for you, not just copied from a textbook.

Plus, if you're in that frustrating perimenopause phase where your periods are playing hide and seek, biomarkers can give you answers. You're not crazy. You're not imagining it. Your FSH is 45, and that explains everything.

At-Home Testing: The Future Is Now

Yes, you can now test some of these hormones at home. Companies are offering finger-prick tests that you can do in your pajamas while watching Netflix. You send the sample back, and boom, you get your results. It's convenient, but here's my advice: use these as a starting point for conversation with your doctor, not as a replacement for professional guidance. Your hormone levels can fluctuate wildly during perimenopause, so one test might show you're menopausal, and another a week later might suggest otherwise. It's like checking the weather forecast in spring. Helpful, but don't cancel your outdoor plans based on one reading.

Custom HRT: Because You're Not a Cookie Cutter

Gone are the days when every menopausal woman got handed the same prescription and sent on her way. Welcome to the era of personalized hormone therapy, where your treatment is as unique as your Netflix recommendations.

What Makes It "Custom"?

Traditional HRT was like buying clothes in sizes small, medium, and large. Custom HRT is like having a tailor measure you and create something that actually fits. Your doctor considers:

- Your specific biomarker levels

- Your symptom severity and type

- Your personal and family health history

- How you respond to initial treatment

- Your lifestyle and preferences

Then they adjust the type of hormones, the dosage, the delivery method, and the timing to match your needs. It's not just about throwing estrogen at the problem anymore.

Delivery Methods: It's Not Just Pills Anymore

The variety of HRT delivery methods now available is honestly impressive:

Patches: Stick one on your skin, and change it once or twice a week. The hormones absorb steadily through your skin, bypassing your liver. Lower risk of blood clots compared to pills.

Gels and Creams: Rub them on your arms or thighs daily. Same benefits as patches, but some women prefer the routine.

Pellets: Tiny hormone pellets inserted under your skin every 3-6 months. Sounds intense, but some women swear by them for steady hormone levels. It's a minor office procedure.

Vaginal Options: Rings, tablets, or creams that treat vaginal symptoms directly without much systemic absorption. Great if dryness is your main complaint.

Oral Pills: Still available and effective, though they have a slightly higher blood clot risk than other methods.

Sprays: Yes, hormone sprays are a thing now. Apply to your forearm daily.

The point is, if one method doesn't work for you or has side effects, you have options. Lots of them.

The Monitoring Part Nobody Talks About

Custom HRT isn't a set-it-and-forget-it situation. Your doctor should be checking in with you regularly, adjusting doses based on how you feel, and sometimes retesting your hormone levels. It's like tuning a guitar. You don't do it once and expect it to stay perfect forever. You adjust as needed.

Most doctors recommend follow-ups at 3 months, then 6 months, then annually once you're stable. Some use symptom tracking apps to monitor your response between visits. The goal is finding your sweet spot, that dose to which symptoms disappear but side effects don't appear.

SERMs and the New Kids on the Block

Okay, now we're getting into the really interesting territory. What if you could get some benefits of estrogen without actually taking estrogen? Enter SERMs and other clever alternatives.

What the Heck Is a SERM?

SERM stands for Selective Estrogen Receptor Modulator. I know, I know, it sounds like something from a sci-fi movie. But here's what it actually means: these medications act like estrogen in some parts of your body (good parts like your bones) while blocking estrogen in other parts (like breast tissue, where too much estrogen can increase cancer risk).

It's like having a really smart bouncer at a club who lets the good guests in and keeps the troublemakers out. Your bones get the estrogen effects they need, but your breast tissue doesn't get the stimulation that might increase cancer risk.

The good news is that you have choices now. Real choices, not just "take this or suffer." The bad news is that more choices mean more complexity. That's where a knowledgeable healthcare provider becomes worth their weight in gold.

What This All Means for You

The landscape of menopause treatment is changing faster than your mood swings during perimenopause. Okay, maybe not that fast, but you get the point. What matters is this: you're not limited to your mother's or grandmother's options anymore.

If your doctor seems unaware of these newer options, don't be afraid to ask about them specifically. Print out recent research if you need to. Bring this section to your appointment. You're not being difficult by asking about biomarker testing or fezolinetant. You're being informed.

If your doctor dismisses your questions or insists that there's only one way to treat menopause, consider getting a second opinion. The science has evolved. Your care should evolve with it.

The future of menopause treatment is personalized, precise, and promising. You don't have to settle for one-size-fits-all care or unnecessary suffering. You deserve treatment that's as unique as your experience of menopause itself.

Your Brain on Menopause: The Neuroprotection Revolution

Let's talk about something that doesn't get nearly enough attention: your brain during menopause. Yes, we've covered brain fog in Chapter Three, but what's emerging now is bigger than forgetting where you put your keys. We're talking about long-term brain health, cognitive decline, and potentially reducing your risk of Alzheimer's disease.

The Critical Window: Timing Is Everything

Here's something your doctor might not have told you: when you start hormone therapy might matter as much as whether you start it at all. This is called the "critical window hypothesis," and it's changing how we think about HRT and brain health.

The basic idea: estrogen has protective effects on your brain, but only if you start it around the time of menopause. Start too late (say, 10 years after your periods stop), and those brain benefits might not materialize. It's like trying to water a plant that's already completely dried out versus watering one that's just starting to wilt.

Research from the Kronos Early Estrogen Prevention Study (KEEPS) showed that women who started HRT within three years of their final period had better cognitive performance and brain structure on MRI scans compared to those who didn't. Their brains literally looked younger (Gleason et al., 2015).

But women who waited years after menopause to start HRT? The benefits were less clear, and in some cases, there might even be risks. The Women's Health Initiative Memory Study found that starting HRT after age 65 actually increased dementia risk. Talk about a plot twist.

What this means for you: If you're considering HRT, sooner is likely better for brain health. This doesn't mean you should panic if you're past that window, but it does mean the conversation about HRT should happen during perimenopause, not a decade later.

Precision Neuroprotection: It's Not Just About Hormones

The exciting frontier in menopause medicine is looking at brain health from multiple angles simultaneously. Think of it as a personalized brain health plan, not just a hormone prescription.

Genetic Testing: Some women carry genetic variants (like APOE4) that affect their Alzheimer's risk and how their brains respond to estrogen. In the future, your doctor might test for these genes before recommending HRT, tailoring your treatment based on your genetic profile. It's like having a roadmap of your brain's vulnerabilities before choosing your route.

Cognitive Training During Transition: Some clinics are now combining HRT with structured cognitive training programs during the menopause transition. The idea is that your brain is particularly plastic (changeable) during this time, so targeted brain exercises might have extra benefits. Early studies are promising, showing improvements in memory and executive function that last beyond the training period.

The Estrogen-Insulin-Brain Connection: Researchers are discovering that estrogen loss doesn't just affect your brain directly. It also affects how your brain uses glucose (sugar) for energy. Some women develop what's called "brain insulin resistance" during menopause, where their brain cells become less efficient at using glucose. This might explain why some women notice cognitive changes even with normal estrogen replacement.

The emerging solution? A combination approach targeting multiple pathways: HRT for hormonal support, plus medications that improve insulin sensitivity (like metformin), plus dietary changes that support brain metabolism. It's precision medicine in action (Mosconi et al., 2017).

The Mediterranean Brain: Diet as Neuroprotection

While we touched on diet in Chapter Five, there's new evidence specifically linking dietary patterns to brain health during menopause. The Mediterranean diet, rich in olive oil, fish, vegetables, and whole grains, appears to offset some of the cognitive effects of menopause.

A 2023 study followed women through their menopause transition and found that those adhering closely to a Mediterranean diet maintained better cognitive function and had less brain shrinkage on MRI. The women eating more processed foods and red meat? Their brains showed accelerated aging.

The mechanism: These foods support healthy blood vessels (crucial for brain health), reduce inflammation, and provide specific nutrients (like omega-3s and polyphenols) that protect brain cells. It's like giving your brain premium fuel during a particularly demanding phase.

Exercise: Your Brain's Best Friend

We've talked about exercise for hot flashes and bone health, but here's another reason to move: it might be the single best thing you can do for your brain during menopause.

Aerobic exercise increases blood flow to your brain, promotes the growth of new brain cells (yes, even in midlife), and boosts levels of brain-derived neurotrophic factor (BDNF), which is basically fertilizer for your neurons. Studies show that women who exercise regularly during menopause maintain better memory and executive function.

The sweet spot appears to be 150 minutes per week of moderate aerobic activity (brisk walking counts), combined with strength training twice weekly. That's it. No marathon running required.

Sleep: The Missing Piece of the Neuroprotection Puzzle

Here's something that connects everything: sleep. Poor sleep during menopause doesn't just make you tired. It might actually increase your risk of cognitive decline and Alzheimer's disease.

During sleep, your brain clears out toxic proteins (including amyloid-beta, associated with Alzheimer's). Chronic sleep disruption from night sweats or insomnia means these proteins build up. Over the years, this accumulation might contribute to cognitive problems.

The neuroprotection strategy here is aggressive treatment of sleep problems. This might mean HRT to stop night sweats, cognitive behavioral therapy for insomnia, treating sleep apnea if present, or all of the above. Your nighttime brain cleaning service needs to run smoothly.

Emerging Therapies: What's on the Horizon

The pipeline of potential neuroprotective treatments for menopausal women is genuinely exciting:

Selective estrogen receptor beta agonists: These would target specific estrogen receptors in the brain without affecting breast or uterine tissue. Think of them as smart bombs for brain protection.

NAD+ precursors: Compounds like nicotinamide riboside that boost cellular energy production are being studied for their potential to support brain metabolism during menopause.

Senolytic drugs: Medications that clear out old, dysfunctional cells (which accumulate faster after menopause) might help preserve brain function. Early trials are underway.

Personalized hormone formulations based on metabolomics: Instead of just measuring hormone levels, future testing might analyze dozens of metabolic markers to create ultra-precise hormone regimens optimized for your brain health.

Your Neuroprotection Action Plan

So what should you do with all this information? Here's a practical approach:

1. Time HRT appropriately: If you're considering hormone therapy, have that conversation early in your menopause transition, not years later.

2. Move your body: Aim for that 150 minutes per week of activity that gets your heart rate up. Your brain will thank you in 20 years.

3. Feed your brain: Shift toward a Mediterranean-style eating pattern. More fish, olive oil, vegetables, and whole grains. Less processed junk.

4. Protect your sleep: Treat sleep problems aggressively. They're not just inconvenient; they're also a brain health issue.

5. Stay mentally active: Challenge your brain regularly with new learning, social engagement, and cognitively demanding activities.

6. Consider genetic testing: If you have a family history of Alzheimer's or strong concerns about cognitive decline, ask your doctor about genetic testing that might inform your treatment decisions.

7. Monitor your metabolic health: Keep your blood sugar, blood pressure, and cholesterol in healthy ranges. What's good for your heart is good for your brain.

The bottom line? The future of menopause care is about more than just surviving hot flashes. It's about optimizing your brain health for the decades ahead. And that future is arriving faster than you think.

From Hot Mess to Hot Empowered: Lisa's Menopause Makeover

Lisa had always been a go-getter. At 49, she was juggling a demanding job in marketing, a busy household with two teenagers, and a beloved garden that was her escape. But then menopause hit, and Lisa felt as if her entire life unraveled overnight.

At first, it was the little things—forgetting appointments or misplacing her keys. Then came the relentless insomnia, where she'd wake up drenched in sweat and be unable to drift back to sleep. Her once-steady weight started climbing despite her best attempts to eat healthily and hit the gym, while her joints ached so much that even walking through the garden felt like climbing Everest. On top of it all, she was snapping at her family and struggling to focus on work.

"I don't even recognize myself," Lisa admitted to her best friend during one of their coffee dates. "I feel like a frumpy, grumpy zombie."

Her breaking point came during a high-stakes work presentation. Mid-sentence, she completely lost her train of thought, stared blankly at her colleagues, and had to excuse herself. She locked herself in the bathroom, tears streaming down her face, wondering how she could continue like this.

That night, Lisa sat down with her laptop and did something she hadn't done before—she researched menopause. For hours, she read stories from women who'd gone through similar struggles and stumbled upon the idea of HRT. She learned about the potential benefits and risks, and for the first time in months, she felt a flicker of hope.

Lisa scheduled an appointment with her doctor, determined to advocate for herself. Sitting in the exam room, she laid it all out: the sleepless nights, the joint pain, the mood swings, the weight gain, and how it was affecting her work and family.

"I've tried everything—exercise, herbal teas, meditation. Nothing's working. I need something more," she said firmly.

Her doctor listened and explained the science behind HRT, dispelling the myths Lisa had heard over the years. They discussed her health history, the potential benefits, and how HRT could help her navigate this stage of life. Feeling educated and empowered, Lisa decided it was the right choice for her.

The changes didn't happen overnight, but within a few weeks, Lisa noticed subtle shifts. First, her sleep improved. No more tossing and turning or waking up soaked in sweat. Then, her energy levels climbed, her joint pain eased, and she found herself back in the garden, pruning and planting without wincing. The weight gain slowed, and she started feeling stronger during her workouts. Most importantly, her brain fog lifted, allowing her to tackle work confidently again.

Six months later, Lisa reflected on her journey. She felt like herself again—no, better than herself. She slept deeply, laughed more, and had the energy to host a family dinner without collapsing in exhaustion afterward. Her confidence returned, and she even got a promotion at work.

Hot Flash Hacks: The Art of Asking the Right Questions

So, you've decided it's time to take control of this wild ride we call menopause. Maybe you've read every article about hot flashes, tried all the herbal teas, and yelled at a random sweater for being too itchy. And now, you're ready to talk to your healthcare provider about HRT. Excellent choice! But before you waltz into the doctor's office, let's ensure you've got a list of questions that will knock off their sensible loafers. Here's your game plan for tackling the HRT conversation with a mix of confidence, curiosity, and maybe just a hint of menopausal sass.

Starting the Conversation: The Icebreaker

Talking about menopause can feel a little awkward. But your doctors have probably heard it all, including someone asking if a hot flash can be blamed for slapping their husband mid-dinner. Here's why this chat is so important: It sets the stage for a partnership with your healthcare provider. When you ask questions, you're not just a passive patient—you're the Beyoncé of your health journey.

Start with:

- "What's your experience of working with women going through menopause?"

- "Can we discuss HRT and whether it might work for me?"

This opens the door to a productive discussion without sounding like you're reading from WebMD in a panic.

Personal Health Assessment: It's All About YOU

What works for your friend Karen (who swears by yoga and green smoothies) might not work for you. That's why personalizing your questions is key.

Try these:

- "What factors should I consider based on my health history?"

- "Do my family history or lifestyle choices affect my suitability for HRT?"

- "What's my risk of developing complications if I start HRT?"

Asking these questions helps your doctor tailor the conversation to you. Plus, it reminds them that you're not just "another patient." You're a queen taking control of her next chapter.

Bringing It All Together

As we wrap up our exploration of HRT, let's take a moment to reflect on the smorgasbord of information we've covered. We've looked into the highs and lows—from the soothing relief HRT offers from those pesky menopausal symptoms to the careful consideration required of its potential risks. While venturing through this maze of options, remember that having open chats with your healthcare providers helps ensure your HRT experience suits your lifestyle and health goals.

We've also peeked into a variety of nonhormonal alternatives, offering paths less traveled by some. Whether adopting healthier lifestyle choices or trying out stress-busting activities, these options remind us that there's more than one way to ride this roller coaster. Supplements and alternative therapies add a sprinkle of magic to the mix, giving you tools to create a menopausal experience as unique as your fingerprint. Remember, you have plenty of people to lean on—so reach out to friends, join support networks, and share your experiences because laughter and camaraderie can change any menopause marathon into the best kind of party.

Chapter Six

"Have You Tried...?": Alternatives Worth Considering

E xploring Nonhormonal Alternatives

Many women seek alternatives to HRT. Let's explore options that embrace a holistic lifestyle and mind-body connection.

Lifestyle Changes

As we have discussed, we begin our wellness tour with lifestyle changes. As they say, you are what you eat, and this is particularly true during menopause. Eating a balanced diet rich in fruits, vegetables, whole grains, and lean proteins can work wonders in keeping pesky symptoms at bay. Think of it as feeding your body the fuel that makes it purr like a kitten rather than growl like an old lawnmower. Alongside diet, regular exercise isn't just about squeezing into those skinny jeans; it's also your champion against menopause symptoms. Exercise releases endorphins, little packets of happiness you can sprinkle throughout the day. Plus, it can help with weight management, bone health, and even mood swings, making it a triple threat against menopausal woes.

Stress management also deserves a gold medal for minimizing menopause symptoms. "Stress less, smile more"— that's the mantra! Simple practices such as deep breathing, meditation, or even taking yourself out on a date (yes, treat yourself!) can reduce stress levels. It might require experimenting to find what suits your style, but investing time in stress-busting activities pays dividends in comfort and peace of mind.

Natural Supplements

Now, let's switch gears to natural supplements. Set aside a cozy evening to read up on black cohosh, evening primrose oil, and other natural supplements that can serve as gentle allies in managing menopause symptoms. However, don't just raid the health food aisle without first doing some detective work. I like a site called Consum erLab.org (they have some free information or a subscription offer). However, if you choose these supplements, doing so thoroughly and consulting healthcare professionals before taking them is imperative, considering they can interact with medications and vary in effectiveness. So, let's dive into supplements as they pertain to menopause. The North American Menopause Society and the American College of Obstetricians and Gynecologists recommend a cautious approach to natural supplements for menopause. They emphasize that while some women may find relief, supplements should not replace evidence-based treatments unless advised by a healthcare professional. For severe symptoms, they often suggest considering hormone therapy or non-hormonal prescription options with a proven safety profile.

A Few Things to Consider About Natural Supplements

1. Lack of Regulation

- Regulatory Oversight: In the United States, the U.S . Food and Drug Administration (FDA), under the Dietary Supplement Health and Education Act (DSHEA) of 1994, regulates natural supplements, including vitamins, minerals, herbs, and other dietary supplements. However, the FDA regulates them less strictly than prescription or over-the-counter (OTC) medications. This means they are not required to undergo the rigorous testing for safety, efficacy, and quality that pharmaceuticals must meet.

- Potential Issues: Some supplements may contain inconsistent dosages, contaminants, or undeclared ingredients. In rare cases, supplements have been found to contain prescription drug analogs or harmful substances.

2. **Risk of Contamination and Purity Issues**

- Heavy Metals and Toxins: Natural supplements, especially those derived from plants, algae, or sea-based sources, can be contaminated with heavy metals (e.g., lead, mercury) or toxins. Use the FDA's TAINTED PRODUCTS MARKETED AS DIETARY SUPPLEMENTS database.

- Pesticides and Additives: Some herbal supplements might also contain pesticide residues or artificial additives.

3. **Interaction with Medications**

- Adverse Interactions: Natural supplements can interact with prescription medications, over-the-counter drugs, and other supplements. For example:

- St. John's Wort can reduce the effectiveness of antidepressants, birth control pills, and blood thinners.

- Ginkgo biloba may increase the risk of bleeding when taken with anticoagulants.

- Calcium and magnesium supplements can interfere with the absorption of certain medications, including antibiotics.

4. Health Risks and Side Effects

- Overdose Risk: Some supplements contain high doses of active ingredients, which can lead to toxicity. For example, excessive vitamin A or D can cause serious health issues.

- Allergic Reactions: Natural supplements can trigger allergic responses, especially those containing herbs, bee products, or marine extracts.

- Harmful Compounds: Some natural supplements contain bioactive compounds that may not be safe for everyone. Kava, for example, causes liver damage, and cardiovascular risks led to ephedra's ban.

5. Efficacy Concerns

- Lack of Evidence: Many natural supplements do not have robust clinical evidence supporting their claimed benefits. While some, like fish oil or probiotics, have substantial research, others rely on anecdotal evidence.

- Placebo Effect: Some perceived benefits may be because of

the placebo effect rather than the supplement's action.

6. Quality and Standardization

- Inconsistent Potency: Because natural products can vary by growing conditions, harvesting methods, and processing techniques, the potency of supplements can fluctuate.

- Third-Party Testing: Look for supplements that independent organizations have tested, such as USP, NSF International, or ConsumerLab.com, which verify the contents and purity.

Popular Natural Supplements

1. Black Cohosh (Actaea racemosa)

Potential Benefits:

- Hot Flashes and Night Sweats: Black cohosh is often used to reduce the frequency and intensity of vasomotor symptoms like hot flashes and night sweats. Some studies suggest mild-to-moderate effectiveness, although results are mixed.

- Mood and Sleep: There is some evidence that black cohosh may help with mood swings and sleep disturbances associated with menopause.

Mechanism of Action:

- The exact mechanism is unclear. Unlike hormone replacement therapy (HRT), black cohosh does not contain phytoestrogen. Instead, it may act on serotonin receptors, which could influence temperature regulation and mood.

Safety and Side Effects:

- Common Side Effects: Generally well-tolerated but may cause stomach upset, rash, or headache.

- Liver Concerns: There have been rare reports of liver damage associated with black cohosh use. It is important to monitor for symptoms of liver issues, such as jaundice or abdominal pain.

- Drug Interactions: Black cohosh may interact with hormone therapies, birth control pills, and medications that affect the liver.

Current Research:

- The North American Menopause Society (NAMS) reports that black cohosh may relieve symptoms for some women but advises against long-term use without medical supervision.

2. Evening Primrose Oil (EPO)

Potential Benefits:

- Menopausal Symptoms: Evening primrose oil is rich in gamma-linolenic acid (GLA), an omega-6 fatty acid that may help reduce breast pain, mood swings, and hot flashes.

- Skin Health: It may also improve dry skin, a common issue during menopause.

Mechanism of Action:

- GLA in evening primrose oil may reduce inflammation and

support hormonal balance. Some believe it might help with prostaglandin production, potentially easing breast tenderness and menstrual symptoms.

Safety and Side Effects:

- Common Side Effects: Mild side effects such as nausea, stomach upset, or headache.

- Blood-Thinning Risk: EPO may have a mild anticoagulant effect, which means it could increase the risk of bleeding, especially when combined with blood-thinning medications (e.g., aspirin, warfarin).

- Seizure Risk: Rarely, EPO may increase the risk of seizures, particularly in individuals with epilepsy or those taking certain antipsychotic medications.

Current Research:

- The evidence for evening primrose oil in managing menopausal symptoms is inconsistent, with some studies showing little to no benefit compared to placebo.

Key Considerations When Using Natural Supplements for Menopause

1. Quality and Purity:

- Choose supplements from brands that undergo third-party testing (e.g., USP, NSF, ConsumerLab.com) to ensure purity, potency, and absence of contaminants.

2. Consultation with Healthcare Provider:

- Always discuss supplement use with your healthcare provider, especially if you are taking prescription medications or have pre-existing health conditions.

3. Monitor for Side Effects:

- Be aware of potential side effects, particularly related to liver health (with black cohosh) and blood clotting (with evening primrose oil).

4. Avoid Combining with Certain Medications:

- These supplements may interact with hormone therapies, anticoagulants, and seizure medications.

Alternative Therapies

Then we have alternative therapies—our next stop on this magical mystery tour of symptom management. Acupuncture might sound like something from Harry Potter's spellbook, but it's an ancient practice that can work wonders by balancing energy flow and reducing hot flashes. Meanwhile, yoga isn't just about molding yourself into a human pretzel; it's about finding balance, harmony, and maybe a giggle or two when attempting the Downward Dog pose. These therapies offer natural ways to ease symptoms while connecting body and mind, providing a holistic approach to wellness.

Finally, we examine the importance of building support networks and community connections. Imagine menopause not as a solo journey through uncharted waters but as a dance party where everyone's learning new steps together. Talking to friends, joining support groups, or sharing experiences online can create a sense of community and belonging. This exchange of stories and strategies often inspires women to look into creative solutions to manage their symptoms while reducing their isolation. After all, a problem shared is a problem halved!

How Acupuncture Works:

- Traditional Chinese Medicine (TCM) Perspective: Acupuncture involves inserting thin needles into specific acupoints on the body to restore energy flow (Qi) and balance the body's systems.

- Western Perspective: Acupuncture stimulates the nervous system, promoting the release of endorphins and other neurochemicals that help regulate mood and reduce pain.

Benefits for Menopausal Symptoms:

- Hot Flashes and Night Sweats: Several studies show that acupuncture may reduce the frequency and severity of vasomotor symptoms.

- Mood and Sleep: Acupuncture can help ease anxiety, depression, and insomnia, which are common during menopause.

- Pain Relief: It may also reduce joint pain and muscle tension, offering relief for menopausal women experiencing aches and stiffness.

Research Highlights:

- A 2021 study published in Menopause: The Journal of the North American Menopause Society found that eight weeks of acupuncture significantly reduced hot flashes and improved quality of life in postmenopausal women.

What to Expect During a Session:

- Sessions typically last 30 to 60 minutes. Many women report feeling relaxed or even energized afterward.

- It is generally considered safe when performed by a licensed acupuncturist and has minimal side effects.

Yoga as a Complementary Therapy for Menopause

How Yoga Helps:

- Mind-Body Connection: Yoga combines physical postures (asanas), breathing exercises (pranayama), and meditation to reduce stress and improve well-being.

- Hormonal Balance: Certain poses may stimulate glands and support hormonal regulation, potentially reducing menopausal symptoms.

Benefits for Menopausal Symptoms:

- Reduces Stress and Anxiety: The mindfulness component of yoga helps manage mood swings and emotional changes.

- Improves Sleep: Relaxation techniques can enhance sleep quality, addressing insomnia and night sweats.

- Enhances Physical Health: Yoga improves flexibility, strength, and bone density, which is beneficial for preventing osteoporosis during menopause.

Recommended Yoga Styles:

- Hatha Yoga: Gentle and beginner-friendly, focusing on breath control and basic postures.

- Restorative Yoga: Emphasizes deep relaxation, which can help with stress management and insomnia.

- Yin Yoga: Involves holding poses for longer periods, targeting deep connective tissues, and promoting joint health.

Practical Tips for Readers:

- Start with short sessions (10-20 minutes) and gradually increase.

- Look for classes or videos that are specifically tailored to menopausal symptoms.

- Incorporate breathing exercises and meditation to support mental health.

Yoga Poses for Menopausal Symptom Relief

1. Cooling Pose for Hot Flashes: "Legs Up the Wall" (Viparita Karani)

- How to Do It: Lie on your back with your legs extended up a wall, forming an L-shape. Arms can rest by your sides or on your abdomen.

- Benefits: Promotes circulation, reduces swelling, and offers a cooling effect that may help with hot flashes.

- Tip: Hold for 5-10 minutes, focusing on deep, relaxed breathing.

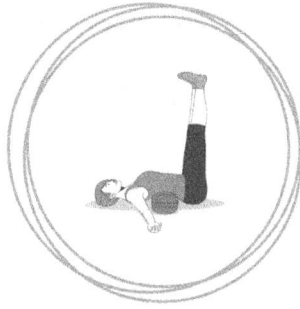

2. Stress and Anxiety Relief: "Child's Pose" (Balasana)

- How to Do It: Sit on your knees, fold forward, and stretch your arms out in front of you with your forehead on the mat.

- Benefits: Provides a sense of safety and grounding, helps calm the mind, and alleviates back and hip pain.

- Tip: Stay in this pose for as long as it feels comfortable, practicing slow, diaphragmatic breathing.

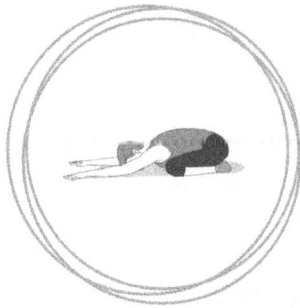

3. Hormonal Balance: "Supported Bridge Pose" (Setu Bandhasana)

- How to Do It: Lie on your back with knees bent and feet flat on the floor. Lift your hips and place a block or pillow under your lower back for support.

- Benefits: Stimulates the thyroid gland, helps with hormonal balance, and relieves tension in the lower back.

- Tip: Hold for 3-5 minutes, breathing deeply and slowly.

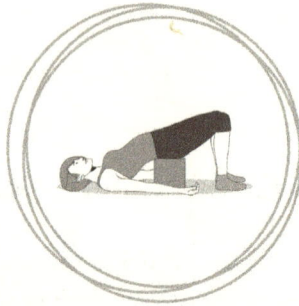

4. Sleep and Relaxation: "Reclined Bound Angle Pose" (Supta Baddha Konasana)

- How to Do It: Lie on your back with the soles of your feet together, knees open to the sides. Support your knees with pillows or blocks for added comfort.

- Benefits: Opens the hips, reduces stress, and can prepare the body for restful sleep.

- Tip: Use a bolster or pillow under your back for additional support and comfort.

Bringing It All Together

Menopause reshapes not only our bodies but also the inner landscape of our minds. By now, you've learned that mood swings, brain fog, and those sudden waves of anxiety aren't signs of weakness—they're messages from a body in transition. When we name what's happening, the shame dissolves, and understanding takes its place.

Emotional balance during this time isn't about forcing calm; it's about cultivating awareness. You've discovered that open conversations—whether with a partner, a friend, or a healthcare professional—transform frustration into connection. You've seen that mindfulness, movement, laughter, and even the right foods can restore a sense of steady ground beneath shifting hormones.

Most of all, this chapter reminds you that menopause isn't the thief of joy; it's the teacher of resilience. Every tear, every laugh, every "Where did I put my glasses?" moment is part of a larger story of growth. When you care for your mind as diligently as your body, you reclaim your sparkle—one mindful breath, one honest conversation, one small act of self-kindness at a time.

So, as you close this chapter, take a deep breath and smile. You're not losing control—you're learning a new rhythm. And just like every woman before you, you'll find your balance again ... perhaps even stronger, wiser, and freer than ever.

Chapter Seven

Between the Sheets: Keeping the Spark Alive

The waves of menopause can feel like starting on a voyage without a map, especially when it comes to its impact on your sex life. Menopause, a natural life stage, brings predictable yet diverse changes. Understanding menopause's changes can be challenging. With menopause, intimacy becomes an adventurous dance, sometimes requiring more than a simple two-step, and bringing with it challenges and revelations alike. This allows us to rediscover and reinvent our personal and shared enjoyment.

Throughout this chapter, we'll dive into the nitty-gritty of how menopause alters sexual health and the intimate connections that accompany it. Expect to uncover the truth behind your fluctuating libido and the infamous duo—vaginal dryness and discomfort—that tends to tag along uninvited. It's a candid exploration, sparing no detail on managing these symptoms while encouraging self-discovery and gratitude for what your body uniquely offers at this stage in life. By spotlighting common emotional shifts and intimacy dynamics, we'll provide insights into maintaining and even enhancing the quality of your sexual experiences.

Communication plays a starring role here; understanding how to foster open, honest dialogue with your partner will ensure you're co-conspirators on this transformative adventure. Embrace curiosity, humor, and a spirited willingness to explore new dimensions of connection as you learn to celebrate the changes, turning what could be seen as obstacles into mere stepping stones toward deeper, more meaningful interactions.

Understanding Physical Changes

By now, you know that menopause marks the end of your menstrual cycles and ushers in hormonal shifts that ripple into your sexual health. Estrogen, progesterone, and testosterone all take a dip, and your body notices. These changes can feel unsettling at first, but here's the truth: they're a normal part of aging, not a problem to fix or a topic to avoid.

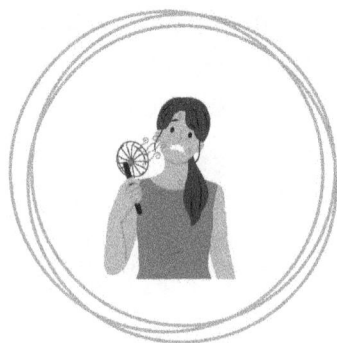

During menopause, many women notice alterations in their libido and overall sexual desire. This fluctuation is mainly because of the shift in hormone levels, which can influence both physical and emotional aspects of sexual health. Reduced estrogen often leads to a decline in sexual interest, although for some, it might spark an unexpected increase. Remember, there's no universal standard for sexual desire during this phase; each person's experience is unique, just like a favorite pair of shoes that somehow still fits perfectly after all these years!

Welcome Physical Symptoms Into the Bedroom

Physical symptoms such as vaginal dryness and discomfort during intercourse are common during menopause. These symptoms occur because plummeting estrogen levels make the vaginal tissue thinner and less lubricated, sometimes causing sexual experiences to be painful. Thankfully, recognizing these symptoms helps you manage them. Over-the-counter vaginal moisturizers or water-based lubricants are what should grace your bedside table. Discussing these changes with a healthcare professional can open doors to tailored treatments.

Beyond the physical, menopause can affect how arousal and orgasm are experienced—aspects that are often overlooked. It's important to understand that your physiological response to sexual stimuli can change, making arousal more challenging and potentially altering your orgasmic responses. These changes don't reflect diminished sexuality but rather a shift manageable through understanding and communication. Emphasizing the importance of open dialogue with your partner ensures both parties are aware of the evolving dynamics of intimacy, helping to create a supportive environment.

Self-Examination and Self-Awareness

Self-Examination and Self-Awareness: Your Power Tools During Menopause embracing self-examination and self-awareness plays a powerful role. Understanding how your body is responding to the changes can empower you to seek regular checkups and develop strategies for enhancing your sexual experiences. Self-discovery isn't just about identifying what's changed—it's about exploring new pathways to pleasure and satisfaction. Think of it as a treasure hunt, but you uncover personal joy and comfort instead of physical gold. Regular visits to your healthcare provider can ensure you're on track and help manage any bothersome symptoms effectively.

Addressing these changes isn't solely the responsibility of one person. If sexual problems arise within a relationship, handling them together can improve satisfaction for both parties. It might be necessary for either partner to seek treatment for their sexual health issues, which can enhance the woman's sexual experiences and function. After all, relationships are team efforts—sometimes, knowing you're both working toward the same goal can make all the difference.

On the brighter side, menopause offers an opportunity to redefine your sexual identity, free from the fear of an unplanned pregnancy, which for some can be pretty liberating. With newfound freedom comes the potential for discovery, allowing you to look into different dimensions of intimacy that weren't possible before. Whether it's trying out new techniques or finding other ways to connect, menopause doesn't have to signify the end of a fulfilling sex life. It's a new chapter, filled with potential for joy and discovery.

Finally, never underestimate the power of humor—a good laugh might just be the best aphrodisiac! Joy and laughter can ease tension and create fond memories that are worth cherishing. It's essential to remain open to learning about yourself, continue communicating with your partner, and embrace this chapter of your life with positivity and curiosity. Humor can be a powerful tool in navigating the challenges of menopause, keeping your spirits high and your relationship strong.

Precision Solutions for Your Sexual Health: Beyond Just Lubricant

Let's be real: when you mention sexual problems during menopause to your doctor, the typical response is predictable. "Try a lubricant. Use a vaginal moisturizer. Maybe some foreplay?" Thanks, doc, but what if the issue goes deeper than just needing more slippery stuff?

The truth is, sexual dysfunction during menopause is complex, involving multiple hormones, neurotransmitters, blood flow, and nerve sensitivity. And just as menopause symptoms vary wildly between women, sexual issues have different root causes for different people. Welcome to precision sexual medicine—where we figure out what's actually broken before trying to fix it.

The Neuroendocrine Orchestra: When the Conductor Goes Missing

Your sexual response isn't just about your genitals. It also involves your brain, hormones, blood vessels, nerves, and how they all communicate. This is called the neuroendocrine system—the connection between your nervous system and your hormones.

During menopause, multiple conductors leave the orchestra:

Estrogen (affects vaginal tissue, lubrication, blood flow)

Testosterone (affects desire, arousal, sensitivity)

DHEA (precursor to both estrogen and testosterone)

Oxytocin (the bonding hormone, also affects arousal)

Dopamine (motivation and pleasure)

Serotonin (mood, but also affects sexual response)

When all these hormones drop or go out of balance, your sexual response system gets confused messages. It's like trying to play a symphony when half the musicians didn't show up.

Diagnosing YOUR Specific Issue: Not All Sexual Problems Are the Same

Before throwing solutions at the problem, let's figure out what your actual problem is. Sexual dysfunction during menopause typically falls into categories:

1. Desire Issues (Low Libido)

You just don't think about sex anymore.

You're not interested even when your partner initiates.

You don't miss sex when you're not having it.

Root causes: Often testosterone deficiency, sometimes thyroid issues, depression, or medication side effects

2. Arousal Difficulties

You want to want sex, but your body doesn't respond.

Minimal genital sensation or blood flow.

Takes forever to get aroused, if at all.

Root causes: Typically, estrogen deficiency affecting genital blood flow and nerve sensitivity, sometimes neurological

3. Orgasm Problems

You have difficulty reaching orgasm or are unable to orgasm.

Your orgasms are weaker or less satisfying than before.

You take much longer to climax.

Root causes: Nerve sensitivity changes, blood flow issues, hormonal imbalances, medications (especially SSRIs)

4. Pain/Discomfort

- Vaginal dryness, burning, or tearing

- Pain with penetration

- Post-sex soreness or irritation

Root causes: Genitourinary syndrome of menopause (GSM), vaginal atrophy from estrogen loss

5. Combination Issues Most women don't fit neatly into one category. You might have low desire AND arousal difficulties, AND some discomfort. Each component needs to be addressed.

Precision Testing: Getting to the Root Cause

To personalize treatment, you need to understand what's going on in your body. Here's what comprehensive sexual health testing might include:

Hormone Panel:

Total and free testosterone: The "desire hormone" that many doctors ignore in women

DHEA-S: Precursor hormone that can be converted to testosterone and estrogen

Estradiol: Affects vaginal tissue health and blood flow

Progesterone: Can affect mood and stress response

SHBG (Sex Hormone Binding Globulin): High levels bind up testosterone, making it unavailable

Thyroid panel: Hypothyroidism kills libido

Prolactin: Elevated levels suppress sexual desire

If you're taking HRT, this testing shows whether your current regimen is optimized for sexual function, not just for stopping hot flashes.

Metabolic Markers:

Fasting glucose and insulin: Insulin resistance affects blood flow and nerve function

Lipid panel: Cholesterol issues affect blood vessel health, including genital blood flow

Vitamin D: Deficiency is linked to sexual dysfunction

B vitamins, especially B12: Important for nerve function and sensitivity

Pelvic Floor Assessment: Sometimes the issue isn't hormonal at all—it's muscular. Tight, weak, or uncoordinated pelvic floor muscles can cause pain and arousal difficulties. A pelvic floor physical therapist can assess this.

Targeted Hormone Interventions: Getting Specific

Once you know your hormone levels, treatment can be precisely tailored.

For Low Desire (Testosterone Deficiency):

Women need testosterone, too! It's crucial for libido, arousal, and orgasm. But most general practitioners don't test women's testosterone or don't know how to treat low levels.

Options:

Testosterone cream (compounded): Applied to the vulva or inner thighs. Dosing is typically 0.5-3 mg daily. Some women notice improvements in 2-3 weeks; full effects take 3-6 months.

Testosterone pellets: Small pellets inserted under the skin every 3-4 months. Provides steady testosterone levels.

DHEA supplementation: Oral DHEA (25-50 mg daily) can boost both estrogen and testosterone. Some women respond very well to this approach.

Intrarosa (prasterone): FDA-approved vaginal DHEA specifically for painful sex. It's converted locally to estrogen and testosterone in vaginal tissue.

Important caveat: Testosterone for women remains controversial and is often prescribed off-label. The FDA hasn't approved testosterone products specifically for women, though research supports its use for menopausal sexual dysfunction. Work with a provider experienced in this area.

For Arousal Issues (Blood Flow and Sensitivity):

Localized Estrogen Therapy:

Vaginal estrogen cream, tablets, or ring: Reverses vaginal atrophy, restores blood flow, improves nerve density

Dosing: Typically used 2-3 times per week after initial daily use

Systemic absorption is minimal, so it's safe for most women, even those who can't take oral HRT

Brands: Estrace cream, Vagifem tablets, Estring ring

Ospemifene (Osphena):

A SERM that specifically targets vaginal tissue

Oral medication (60mg daily)

Improves vaginal cell health, lubrication, and reduces pain

Takes 8-12 weeks for full effect

PT-141 (Bremelanotide):

An FDA-approved injection for hypoactive sexual desire disorder

Works on the central nervous system to increase desire and arousal

Self-injected in the abdomen or thigh 45 minutes before anticipated sexual activity

Acts on melanocortin receptors in the brain (completely different mechanism from hormones)

Common side effects: nausea (in about 40% of users), flushing

This is genuinely new and different—it's not a hormone (Clayton et al., 2016)

The Neurotransmitter Approach for Orgasm Difficulties:

Sometimes the issue isn't hormones—it's neurotransmitters. SSRIs (antidepressants) are notorious for causing orgasm difficulties. If you're on an SSRI for mood or hot flashes, this might be your culprit.

Options:

Switch antidepressants: Bupropion (Wellbutrin) doesn't cause sexual side effects and might even improve libido

Add bupropion to your current SSRI: This can counteract sexual side effects

Sildenafil (Viagra): Yes, it works for some women by increasing blood flow. It's used off-label for female sexual dysfunction (Nurnberg et al., 2008)

Oxytocin nasal spray: Some compounding pharmacies offer this. Oxytocin can enhance arousal and orgasm intensity

For Pain and Vaginal Atrophy:

This is probably the most treatable aspect of menopausal sexual dysfunction, yet many women suffer unnecessarily.

The Gold Standard:

Vaginal estrogen: Restores tissue thickness, elasticity, lubrication, and pH balance. Most women see dramatic improvement within 4-8 weeks.

New Options:

Vaginal laser therapy (MonaLisa Touch, FemTouch): Uses fractional CO2 laser to stimulate collagen production and tissue regeneration. Studies show significant improvements in vaginal health and sexual function. Typically, 3 treatments spaced 4-6 weeks apart, with annual maintenance.

Radiofrequency therapy (ThermiVa): Similar concept to laser—stimulates tissue regeneration and tightening. Non-invasive.

Platelet-Rich Plasma (PRP) injections (O-Shot): Your own blood is processed to concentrate growth factors, then injected into the clitoris and vaginal walls. Controversial and expensive, but some women report improvements in sensitivity and orgasm.

Combination Approaches: Most women get the best results from combining treatments:

- Vaginal estrogen + testosterone cream

- HRT + vaginal laser therapy + testosterone

- Testosterone + PT-141 for special occasions

- DHEA + pelvic floor therapy

The Genetic Component: Why Some Treatments Work Better for You

Emerging research shows that genetic variants affect sexual function and treatment response:

AR (Androgen Receptor) Gene: Variations affect how sensitive your tissues are to testosterone. Some women have androgen receptors that don't respond well to normal testosterone levels—they might need higher doses or benefit less from testosterone therapy.

ESR1 (Estrogen Receptor Alpha): Variants affect vaginal tissue response to estrogen. Some women need higher doses of vaginal estrogen to see improvements.

Dopamine Receptor Genes (DRD2, DRD4): Affect motivation, pleasure, and sexual desire. Variants might predict who responds to dopamine-enhancing treatments.

Currently, this testing isn't standard, but some functional medicine practitioners offer it. In 5-10 years, expect genetic testing to guide sexual health treatment decisions just like it's beginning to guide psychiatric medication selection.

Creating Your Personalized Sexual Health Plan

Here's a practical approach to figuring out what will work for you:

Step 1: Identify Your Primary Issue(s)

- Desire, arousal, orgasm, pain, or combination?

- How long has this been going on?

- Did it start with menopause or perimenopause?

Step 2: Get Comprehensive Testing

- Hormone panel (especially testosterone, estradiol, DHEA)

- Metabolic markers

- Review current medications for sexual side effects

Step 3: Start with First-Line Treatments

- **For pain/dryness:** Vaginal estrogen (try for 8-12 weeks)

- **For low desire:** Testosterone therapy trial (3-6 months to assess)

- **For arousal issues:** Combine vaginal estrogen with systemic HRT if appropriate

Step 4: Add Targeted Interventions

- Not improving? Consider PT-141, sildenafil, or oxytocin

- Pelvic floor therapy if muscle issues are present

- Vaginal laser or radiofrequency if estrogen alone isn't enough

Step 5: Optimize and Maintain

Once you find what works, stick with it. Reassess every 6-12 months and adjust doses or treatments as needed.

What About "Natural" Options?

Let's address the supplements and herbs marketed for sexual health:

Maca root: Some evidence for improving sexual desire. Doses of 1,500-3,000mg daily. Worth trying, though effects are modest (Shin et al., 2010).

L-arginine: Amino acid that improves blood flow. Studies show mixed results, but some women report improvements in arousal. Typical dose: 3-5 grams daily.

Ginkgo biloba: Might improve blood flow and counteract SSRI-induced sexual dysfunction. Evidence is weak.

Fenugreek: Some studies show increases in sexual desire and arousal. Typical dose: 600mg daily.

The reality: Natural supplements can help mild symptoms but rarely solve significant sexual dysfunction. They're worth trying, especially if you want to avoid medications, but set realistic expectations.

The Psychological Component: When It's Not Just Physical

Sometimes sexual issues during menopause are partly or entirely psychological:

- Relationship problems that predate menopause

- Body image concerns

- Stress and mental load

- History of sexual trauma

- Depression or anxiety

Even when the root cause is hormonal, the psychological impact compounds the problem. You try to have sex, but it doesn't work or hurts, so you avoid it, which creates tension, which makes the problem worse.

Sex therapy with a certified sex therapist (AASECT-certified) can be incredibly helpful, either alone or combined with medical treatments. Cognitive behavioral therapy specifically for sexual dysfunction has strong research support.

Practical Scripts: Talking to Your Doctor

Some doctors are uncomfortable discussing female sexual health. Here are scripts to make the conversation easier:

Opening: "I'm experiencing changes in my sexual function since menopause, and I'd like to explore treatment options beyond just using lubricant."

If they seem dismissive: "I understand sexual changes are common in menopause, but they're significantly affecting my quality of life and relationship. I'd like to do comprehensive hormone testing, including testosterone, DHEA, and thyroid levels."

If they say "testosterone isn't FDA-approved for women": "I understand it's off-label, but research supports its use for menopausal sexual dysfunction. I'd like to try it with proper monitoring. Can you prescribe it, or should I see a specialist who does?"

If they have no experience with this: "Can you refer me to a menopause specialist or sexual medicine specialist who has experience treating these issues?"

The Bottom Line on Sexual Health

Sexual function matters. It's not frivolous or selfish to want a satisfying sex life in midlife and beyond. And it's not something you have to accept as "just part of aging."

Precision approaches to sexual health during menopause involve:

- Identifying your specific type of dysfunction

- Testing to understand the root causes

- Targeted treatments based on your biology

- Combination approaches when needed

- Addressing both physical and psychological components

The tools exist. The treatments work. You just need to find providers who take sexual health seriously and are willing to go beyond "try a lubricant."

Your sexuality doesn't end at menopause. It just needs a different approach.

Communicating With Your Partner

It's important to remember that open dialogue with your partner is like securing your seat belt—necessary for a safer journey through the twists of menopause. Expressing your feelings openly can create an emotional connection, paving the way for realistic expectations. Expressing what you're going through helps your partner understand, making them more likely to offer empathy and support. Your partner is your copilot—they need to know when turbulence hits. This open dialogue can reassure you that you're not alone on this journey.

It's Time to Talk About the Changes

Letting your partner know about your menopause symptoms isn't just polite; consider it your personal public service announcement that brings understanding and fosters support. You wouldn't let your copilot fly blind, would you? By educating your partner about how menopause might affect your sexual health, you equip them to better support you, which can strengthen your relationship and deepen your bond. After all, no one wants their favorite teammate to feel left out of the game plan!

Let's discuss what's really bothering us: fear and embarrassment. It's okay to feel awkward sometimes, but normalizing these discussions can make a difference. Humor is your secret weapon here, as a little laughter can ease discomfort and make potentially sensitive topics a bit lighter. Who knew "menopause humor" could become a genre of its own? Sharing a laugh doesn't just break the ice—it melts it entirely, making way for genuine conversations free from stigma or shame.

Setting Healthy Boundaries

One key ingredient to a healthy dialogue is setting mutual boundaries that ensure trust and emotional safety. No one enjoys feeling exposed without warning, so consider setting boundaries as putting up a mindful fence around your shared emotional garden. Discussing and agreeing on what's comfortable helps establish a foundation of trust. And remember, boundaries aren't etched in stone; revisiting them over time is important for maintaining dynamic communication. Changes may occur, and if you treat boundaries like software updates, you'll keep your connection fresh and secure.

Next, let's address a common scenario: conversations after a revealing episode of night sweats. You wake up drenched, feeling as if you've run a marathon in your sleep. Instead of letting this become an unspoken source of stress, bring it into conversation with humor and openness: "Who needs a gym membership with workouts like last night, right?" This approach invites your partner to share in the experience, leading to mutual support rather than frustration.

Similarly, discussing the adjustments needed for physical comfort during intimacy shouldn't feel like ordering a complicated coffee. Be clear and patient, allowing your partner to understand and engage in finding solutions. Maybe experimenting with different positions or using specifically designed lubricants could help. Such changes don't have to be hurdles but can be approached as opportunities for exploration, making intimacy less about perfection and more about pleasure.

Enhancing Intimacy and Connection

Just because menopause has entered your life doesn't mean you're closing the chapter on intimacy. In fact, it's an opportunity to rewrite the story of your sexual life, adding elements that build deeper connections and revitalize joy. Here, we delve into actionable tips for maintaining and enhancing intimacy during menopause because menopause isn't the end; it's a transformation.

Exploring new activities can strengthen bonds that extend beyond physical intimacy. Consider this time in your life as an invitation to rediscover the simple joys you and your partner can share. Try engaging in hobbies or activities neither of you has explored before—maybe consider taking up dance lessons, cooking classes, or simply hiking together. The key is to break free from routine and embrace novelty. These adventures add excitement and offer opportunities to learn about each other's evolving interests.

Prioritizing your emotional connection is essential for nurturing a relationship built on understanding, which will directly benefit your sexual health. Open and honest communication forms the foundation of this emotional closeness. Share your thoughts, fears, and desires with your partner, creating a space where you both feel heard and valued. Setting boundaries is also necessary here; ensure that whatever makes you uncomfortable is communicated gently but firmly. This mutual respect creates an environment where intimacy can flourish naturally.

Touch and Affection

Nonsexual physical affection, such as cuddling, plays a role in maintaining intimacy, offering warmth and comfort that extends foreplay beyond conventional approaches. Regularly hugging, holding hands, or simply lying close to each other without any expectations helps sustain your affectionate bond. This type of touch reassures both partners of your commitment to each other, even when traditional notions of sexual activity might be changing.

Diving into creative exploration in sexual expression can improve your satisfaction by allowing open experimentation with your desires. Don't shy away from discussing fantasies or trying out new ways of expressing yourselves sexually. Introduce playful elements such as role-playing or use tools such as erotic literature or adult toys. This phase of life encourages self-discovery and a redefinition of pleasure, breaking away from past restrictions. Remember, it's not about comparison or performance; it's about finding what brings mutual enjoyment. If any of this is making you or your partner squirm in your seat, consider a professional sex therapist. Yes, that is a thing, and there are therapists out there who have studied how to help couples have a fulfilling, intimate relationship.

When considering these tips, try integrating small changes that can have substantial impacts. For example, setting aside planned intimacy dates ensures you prioritize time for just the two of you within your bustling schedules; it's about intention rather than spontaneity. Build anticipation by sharing flirtatious messages throughout the day, setting a positive tone in the lead-up to your date night.

Some might wonder if less frequent sex means something negative; however, it's essential to accept that everyone's experience is unique, and less sex is perfectly okay if that's the new normal for you. What matters most is the quality of the moments shared and the genuine connection maintained, regardless of how often intercourse occurs. Embracing these changes with acceptance and humor can ease the pressure and augment your intimacy in unexpected ways.

Addressing specific menopausal symptoms that affect intimacy shouldn't be overlooked. Products like lubricants and moisturizers ease the discomfort associated with vaginal dryness, making intercourse more enjoyable. Couple these solutions with discussions with healthcare providers to look into medical treatments if necessary.

Resources for Sexual Health Support

Handling the messiness of menopause and its effect on your sexual health is like setting off on a new adventure—one that might seem overwhelming at first. Still, it offers countless opportunities for growth and discovery. Consulting medical professionals becomes like having a personalized road map during this phase. These experts can provide insights tailored just for you, helping with informed decisions about managing menopausal symptoms. Whether addressing hormonal changes or exploring treatment options, a healthcare provider can guide you through this journey, ensuring you're equipped with the right tools to maintain your desired quality of life. Remember, it's essential to seek specialists with specific menopausal expertise since not every doctor is fully versed in its intricacies.

Now, let's talk more about therapies and counseling. Think of these as the supportive cheerleaders along your path, addressing any psychological hurdles that may arise. Counseling offers a safe space to share experiences and gain perspective. In contrast, group therapies or individual counseling sessions can help break down psychological barriers that might otherwise impede intimacy, providing invaluable emotional support.

Educational resources are indispensable for those seeking truth amid the myths surrounding menopause. Books, forums, and workshops offer facts and information, clearing the fog of misconceptions. Through these mediums, you can engage directly with experts and peers, ask questions, and build a knowledge base that demystifies menopause. Understanding the biological shifts within your body ease your anxiety and enable you to accept the changes with confidence and curiosity.

Last, let's add laughter into the mix. Menopause can be challenging, but laughter is an excellent medicine. Shared laughter eases the transition's somberness. Humor opens the door to open communication, creating a comfortable environment where everyone feels free to express their needs and desires.

Bringing It All Together

As you navigate menopause, remember: change is inevitable, but it's natural—not something to fear. By understanding your body's responses and exploring new ways to maintain intimacy, you can move through this transition with confidence. You've learned about hormonal impacts, symptom management, and partner communication—consider it your troubleshooting guide for the body's natural "upgrades."

This isn't just about coping; it's about discovering new opportunities for connection and joy. Menopause doesn't end a satisfying sex life—it's a chance to redefine it on your terms. Whether that means laughing through hot flashes or exploring new adventures together, there's room for creativity. Embrace the freedom of this phase: no worry about unplanned pregnancy, no more time and energy spent on monthly cycles and period supplies.

You're not just surviving menopause—you're thriving through it, turning potential obstacles into opportunities for a more fulfilling intimate life. Celebrate this chapter with curiosity and humor, because aging gracefully means embracing change with a light heart.

Chapter Eight

Your Menopause Tribe: Nobody Sweats Alone

B uilding a support network is like sewing a friendship quilt during menopause; each patch represents the unique stories and experiences of women who stitch together a comforting blanket of camaraderie despite the hot flashes and mood swings. This phase of life can often feel like you're auditioning for the lead role in *The Hot Flash Chronicles*. Instead, imagine standing on a vast stage teeming with women who totally get it and are ready to swap their best survival tips. Whether it's bonding over baffling new symptoms or sharing secrets to outwit insomnia, menopause becomes more colorful and less intimidating with a community by your side.

In this chapter, we'll investigate how to fortify your life's patchwork of new connections, offering local and digital avenues to widen your circle of support. Diverse options cater to all interests, from social gatherings to online communities. So, grab a cozy seat and build a support network that feels like home, one unique story at a time.

Building a Support Network

Menopause can be a challenging time, but a strong support network can make all the difference. Feelings of isolation often accompany this transition, so sharing stories during this time can work wonders by fostering connections and understanding between women facing similar experiences. It's incredible how sharing personal accounts can create a sense of belonging and empathy. Suddenly, you're part of a club where the other members genuinely get what you're going through. These shared narratives reduce isolation. You're not just part of a club. You're part of a supportive community that accepts you for who you are.

Local Support Groups

Now, how do you find or create these valuable connections? Local support groups offer an excellent starting point. They bring people together face-to-face and provide a safe space for open discussion and camaraderie. These interactions nurture trust and solidarity as the participants share laughter, tears, and everything in between.

Establishing such a group might sound daunting, but trust me—it's easier than you think. Begin by tapping into existing local resources such as community centers, libraries, or healthcare facilities, which often have bulletin boards or newsletters. Social media is also a fantastic tool for spreading the word about setting up a new group. Remember, it's about creating a welcoming environment where everyone feels comfortable taking part. Consistency in meeting times and having a clear agenda can help your group take root and thrive.

Healthcare Providers

Healthcare providers can play an invaluable role in building your support network. Many professionals are eager to facilitate workshops and discussions tailored to your needs, enhancing understanding and empowerment during menopause. Attending engaging sessions led by experts can help address your concerns and provide evidence-based insights. By collaborating with healthcare workers, you gain access to knowledge that empowers you to handle menopause with confidence. The empowerment that comes from gaining knowledge and insights can make you feel more confident and capable of managing your menopause journey.

Check with your doctor or local wellness clinics to see if they host any events or workshops. Some may even offer CBT or other mental health support specifically designed for menopausal symptoms. This blend of medical expertise and peer interaction can be an enormous help.

Let's not forget community events centered on menopause education. Taking part in such activities isn't just informative—it's also a chance to break down societal stigmas around menopause. Engaging in workshops or seminars also opens doors to new friendships while promoting informed dialogues. You can exchange tips and tricks on managing symptoms or discuss how different cultures perceive menopause. These interactions build both understanding and acceptance.

It could be as simple as attending a local health fair or webinar on women's health issues. Look for talks or panels at your local community center or online. Such events can enhance your knowledge while allowing you to meet others in a fun and relaxed setting.

Stories from Women Who've Been There

Within menopause, there's a certain power in stories—the kind that makes you nod along as if someone just read your mind. Sharing authentic narratives from women who've lived through this transition brings comfort and understanding. Let's look at some of these narratives and how they can soothe and teach us about this transformative phase.

Take Beth, for instance. Unexpected hot flashes plagued her, even while driving or in a blizzard. Desperate for relief, Beth turned to yoga. At first, it felt like a cruel joke. Holding poses like a downward dog while feeling like a human bonfire wasn't her idea of serenity. But over time, something clicked. The slow stretches eased her tension, the deep breathing calmed her mind, and the hot flashes didn't feel as volcanic. Beth found her groove, paired with herbal teas, which she swore tasted of hay but somehow worked. She called it her "Zen and tonic" routine and recommended it to anyone listening.

Then there's Krista, who decided enough was enough after one particularly frustrating day of forgetting not one but three appointments. Instead of hiding her struggles, she joined a local menopause support group. What she found there was better than therapy—it was laughter. The group didn't just share tips; they shared stories, including when one woman accidentally brought her husband's orthopedic socks to yoga class or another mistook her hot flash for a fever and took three rapid COVID tests in an hour. Krista found comfort in the humor and camaraderie, and her weekly group became her sanctuary. She walked out of each meeting feeling less alone and more equipped to face the challenges of menopause.

Little Victories, Big Wins

It's not just the Beths and Kristas of the world who inspire. Nancy also conquered insomnia with a genius combination of bamboo sheets and a cooler thermostat. After months of tossing and turning in her sweat-soaked sheets, she'd finally Googled "best sheets for night sweats" at 3:00 a.m. and discovered bamboo. "They're like sleeping in an igloo," Nancy said, showing off her newly found glow after getting some rest. She even started keeping a fan at the foot of her bed, creating what she calls her "DIY Arctic tundra."

And we also have Bea, who turned to watercolor painting to tackle her anxiety. Bea had always been a perfectionist, so painting felt intimidating at first. However, she gave it a whirl when a friend gifted her a watercolor set. Surprisingly, she found solace in the soft brushstrokes and flowing colors. Painting became her meditation—a place where she could let go of the tension and simply *be*. Over time, her anxiety lessened, and her walls filled with whimsical landscapes and abstract sunsets. "It's not about being good at painting," Bea often says. "It's about letting the paint flow, just like life."

Shared Wisdom, Unshakable Connection

What ties these stories together isn't just the solutions. Its the connection they create. Each woman's journey is uniquely hers, but by sharing their struggles and successes, they light the way for others. Beth's yoga and tea routine, Krista's laughter-filled support group, Nancy's bamboo sheets, and Bea's watercolor masterpieces became lifelines for someone else. These moments of solidarity remind us that menopause doesn't have to be a lonely, isolating journey. We can instead share an adventure, celebrating each other's small victories, laughing at life's absurdities, and swapping tips to make life easier.

Because it's not about avoiding the storm—it's about finding the community that helps you dance in the rain (or at least sweat through it).

Anonymity and Privacy

A critical component of sharing stories is addressing privacy concerns. Some of us might feel apprehensive about opening up. That's perfectly normal. For this reason, providing options for anonymity within storytelling can be important. Think of it like attending a masquerade ball, where you can share your tale without revealing your identity. It's about creating an atmosphere of trust where you can exchange experiences openly without fear of judgment or exposure. Creating this environment benefits the storyteller and the listener, who can absorb these insights comfortably. So your story matters, and you can choose how and when to share it. These anonymous stories still carry profound power to enlighten and empower.

Remain Inclusive

However, let's not stop there. Inclusivity is paramount when sharing women's stories, and considering race, culture, and socioeconomic background further enriches these accounts. Hearing from Marisol, who's managing menopause alongside cultural expectations that prioritize silence over speaking out, and from Amy, whose access to healthcare differs significantly because of her socioeconomic circumstances, gives us a fuller, richer understanding of menopause as a collective experience. A focus on diversity brings forward voices that might otherwise go unheard, encouraging a dialogue that respects and celebrates the broad spectrum of womanhood. It's about lifting one another and ensuring no voice is left behind.

Let's also consider the current research underlining the diversity of menopause experiences. A study underscores how factors such as employment conditions, culture, and life course elements shape the menopause experience at work. Moreover, a recent report provides insight into the global experiences of women during menopause, recognizing how culture, access to healthcare, and mental health influence their journeys (Menopause Foundation of Canada, 2024).

Online Communities and Resources

In today's digitally connected world, women navigating menopause find themselves with abundant online resources. These platforms provide information and create spaces for support and shared experiences that transcend borders and boundaries. It all starts with the community-focused groups on social media sites like Facebook and Reddit, which offer virtual gatherings where you can throw in your two cents' worth or sit back and quietly absorb wisdom from fellow menopause warriors. These groups are full of advice, humor, and camaraderie, offering solace and diverse perspectives without needing a passport. Such engagement can help alleviate feelings of isolation by connecting you with others who truly understand what you're going through, allowing shared experiences to become a source of relief.

Webinars and Online Workshops

As we dive deeper into the digital landscape, it becomes clear that learning about menopause isn't limited to group discussions. Enter webinars and online workshops—your personal interactive classrooms, available right from the comfort of your home. Experts in women's health host these sessions, providing insights that empower you to make informed decisions about your well-being. It doesn't matter if you're a morning person or a night owl, as these resources fit into any schedule, making continuous learning as easy as brewing a cup of soothing herbal tea. A well-chosen webinar can be enlightening and conversational, striking the right balance between comprehensive education and the encouragement needed to tackle any new phase head-on.

Blogs and Podcasts

For those who prefer to soak up knowledge during their commute or while folding laundry, blogs, and podcasts offer bite-sized morsels of wisdom. The beauty of this diverse content lies in its adaptability. Whether you're a visual learner or someone who learns best via auditory means, there's something for everyone. Some popular blogs offer firsthand accounts from women who've trekked the menopausal path before you, complete with tips and anecdotal experiences that resonate profoundly personally. Meanwhile, podcasts serve up engaging discussions and interviews with health experts, delivering insights with a relatable human touch. This approach aids understanding and facilitates a comforting connection with women globally, one episode at a time.

Telehealth Services

Beyond educational content, telehealth services and virtual support offer invaluable aid when personalized care is required. In a world where visiting clinics might seem daunting, accessing healthcare professionals online opens doors to specialized knowledge without you having to leave your house. Online consultations allow for tailored advice that addresses unique symptoms or concerns relevant to your experience. These digital doctor visits break down geographical barriers, ensuring expert care is within reach no matter where you reside. Moreover, virtual counseling sessions provide emotional support, encouraging conversations that build resilience and empowerment during this transformative period.

In exploring these diverse resources, remember that engaging with technology should be intuitive and stress-free. Virtual interaction may feel unfamiliar at first, but it's surprisingly comfortable once you adapt.

The digital world offers options to strengthen your approach to menopause—from supportive groups to personalized telehealth consultations. Each platform can be a helpful friend, ready to lend a listening ear or insightful advice whenever needed. By embracing these opportunities, you educate yourself and actively participate in a vibrant community. Remember, while each woman's path through menopause is unique, the digital tools available today ensure no one has to walk it alone.

Menopause can affect women of different races and ethnicities differently from a physiological perspective. Research has shown that there are differences in the timing, symptoms, and health impacts of menopause among racial and ethnic groups. *Note:* While findings are not universally applicable, here are a few facts to consider: (Avis, N. E., Crawford, S. L., & Greendale, G.,2021).

Category	African American Women	Latina Women	Caucasian Women	Asian Women
Age at Menopause	Earlier (avg. 49 years)	Earlier (similar to African American)	Average (avg. 51 years)	Later (avg. 51-52 years)
Hot Flashes & Vasomotor Symptoms	More frequent and severe; night sweats last up to 10+ years	Moderate frequency	Moderate frequency	Fewer hot flashes, particularly Japanese and Chinese descent
Muscle & Joint Pain	Higher rates	Higher rates	Moderate rates	Lower rates
Bone Health	Higher bone density, lower osteoporosis risk, but worse outcomes when osteoporosis develops	Higher bone density, lower osteoporosis risk	Higher risk of osteoporosis and fractures	Higher risk of osteoporosis and fractures
Cardiovascular Risk	Higher risk; menopause affects lipid profiles & blood pressure significantly	Moderate to higher risk	Moderate risk; increased cholesterol	Moderate risk; increased cholesterol
Weight & Metabolic Changes	More likely to gain weight, increased risk of metabolic syndrome and diabetes	More likely to gain weight, increased risk of metabolic syndrome and diabetes	Moderate weight gain	Less weight gain overall, but may experience increased abdominal fat
Hormone Levels	Higher estradiol and FSH during transition	Varies	Moderate levels	Lower hormone levels
Duration of Transition	Longer perimenopause	Moderate duration	Shorter transition	Shorter transition and menopausal phase

Bringing It All Together

Ah, the power of connection! We've journeyed through the importance of building a community, sharing experiences during menopause, and forming an unbreakable support team against life's unexpected messes. You're not alone in this mess of chin hairs and brain fog. Instead, you're part of a vibrant tribe full of shared laughter and stories that make you nod and think, *Wow, she really gets me.* Whether it's a local gathering where camaraderie blooms over coffee or an online chat where empathy spans continents, these moments blend a mix of understanding and acceptance. Who knew that swapping tales and tips could feel like finding hidden treasures in your own backyard?

And let's talk about how accessible all this is! From cozy chats at community centers to scrolling through online forums in your pajamas, there are countless ways to find your people and trade those golden nuggets of wisdom. Maybe you'll start attending workshops led by experts or even host your own spirited meeting. Who says a little fun can't accompany serious topics? The idea is to create an inviting space where every voice feels valued and heard, whether quirky or quiet.

As you enjoy these shared stories, know that each adds color to our shared canvas, illustrating a path that's anything but solitary. So go ahead, reach out, connect, and sprinkle a bit of humor along the way—it's the perfect way to lift spirits and share strength.

Chapter Nine

Speak Up, Buttercup: Becoming Your Own Menopause Advocate

A dvocating for yourself is like becoming the CEO of your own health and menopause path. Picture this: you're the star of an epic adventure movie where hot flashes and sleepless nights are the villains. Armed with knowledge, preparation, and a smattering of comedy, you're ready to conquer every obstacle in your path. It's an empowering and entertaining process that promises to tackle your symptoms and strengthen your overall well-being.

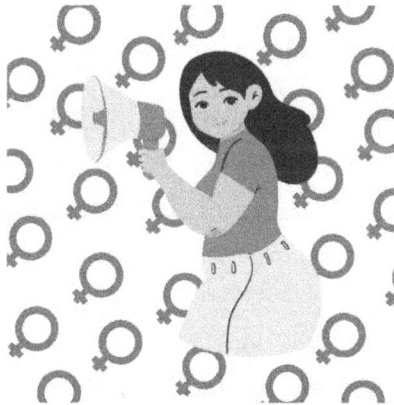

As you step into this role, you'll find that taking charge doesn't mean being confrontational, but clear and confident. It's about confidently translating bodily cues into words so doctors can work with you as allies, solving each quirky mystery menopause throws your way.

In this chapter, we'll explore how to communicate effectively with healthcare providers, ensuring you're never lost in translation during appointments filled with medical jargon and time constraints. Tips empower you to advocate for your health, from organizing records to asking effective questions. Get ready to embrace the art of being your best champion, where your voice becomes your most powerful ally in steering through this life stage on your terms.

Communicating Effectively with Healthcare Providers

Understanding your health concerns is vital to addressing your needs during medical appointments. Whether you're dealing with hot flashes, sleep disturbances, or emotional shifts, it's crucial to appreciate what's happening within your body. Think of this self-awareness as having a secret decoder ring for your health. When you can articulate exactly what you're experiencing, you're in a position to communicate effectively with your healthcare provider.

Being assertive in explaining your symptoms and expressing your preferences plays a significant role in achieving better healthcare outcomes. This doesn't mean throwing on a cape and adopting a superhero stance in front of your doctor. Instead, it's about being confident and unreserved when discussing your symptoms. For instance, if night sweats are leaving you drenched and sleepless, don't shy away from emphasizing their severity and frequency. This direct approach helps create a vivid picture of your daily struggles, allowing for solutions tailored to your specific needs. Remember, assertiveness isn't about speaking loudly; it's about speaking clearly and sincerely.

Building trust with doctors allows for a fruitful dialogue about fears or misconceptions. Partner with your doctor to solve "The Menopausal Mysteries"—openly exploring treatments and lifestyle changes. Mutual respect and honesty between you and your healthcare provider can dismantle any wall of misunderstanding and create space for conversations that address even your most uncomfortable questions. There needs to be a safe environment in which patients can openly discuss their fears about hormone therapies or alternative treatments without judgment or dismissal.

Organized Health Records

These are like treasure maps, guiding your healthcare provider through the intricate landscape of your medical history. Your health records include medication lists, past procedures, and family medical history, each serving as an invaluable clue to the most effective treatment. Organizing and updating these documents will ensure nothing slips through the cracks during your appointments. Visualize yourself walking into the doctor's office with a neatly arranged binder of your health history—a tangible reminder of who you are and what you've endured. This preparation empowers you, facilitating a comprehensive discussion and helping the doctor understand your unique circumstances holistically.

Organizing your health records also signals to healthcare providers that you're serious about your health. It shows preparedness, which is often reciprocated by the provider's attention to detail and thoroughness during consultations. While this might sound like extra homework, think of it as carving out time to invest in your well-being. Each page you organize represents an added layer of clarity of communication between you and your healthcare provider.

Proper Tools and Advocacy

Being smack-dab in the middle of menopause requires proper tools and steadfast advocacy. One effective strategy is to prepare specific questions or topics to discuss during appointments. Having a list means you won't forget important points within the flurry of medical jargon or the time constraints often present in clinical settings. You can include questions about alternative therapies or the side effects of certain medications. Planning your questions beforehand makes sure you don't miss anything important. This allows for focused conversations that give you the best information.

Assertiveness paired with preparation isn't just about ticking off boxes; it reassures you that you are advocating effectively for your health. Beyond building trust and improving your healthcare interactions, these steps reinforce your command over your health narrative. By being vocal and organized, you're essentially saying, "I'm the protagonist here, leading my health story."

Sometimes, being the protagonist also involves knowing when to seek further clarification if something isn't clear. If a prescribed treatment plan seems vague or overwhelming, ask for more straightforward explanations or more information. A clear understanding of your treatment options fosters informed decision-making, allowing you to weigh benefits against potential risks confidently.

Let's not overlook the power of humor and lightheartedness amid the stress of medical appointments. A little laughter might be the icebreaker you need to shift the conversation from strictly medical to more personal, strengthening your connection with your healthcare provider. After all, laughter breaks barriers, making patients and doctors more comfortable and open.

Understanding Your Healthcare Rights

Advocating for yourself is a superpower that every woman should harness in the whirlwind of navigating menopause. One aspect of empowerment lies in understanding your healthcare rights, which can transform daunting medical landscapes into safer and more supportive environments.

First, understand your rights as a patient. Much like a trusty umbrella on a rainy day, these rights shield us from potential pitfalls in medical care. Familiarizing yourself with these rights doesn't just offer protection; it builds trust with your healthcare providers. Ever notice how a comprehensive menu at a restaurant gives you confidence in the chef? Similarly, knowing your patient's rights assures you that your treatment is ethical. This familiarity allows you to engage with healthcare professionals confidently, creating an atmosphere where both parties work together toward the best possible outcome.

1. The Right to Informed Consent

- You have the right to understand the benefits, risks, and alternatives of any medical treatment or procedure.

- This means being fully informed before agreeing to hormone therapy, medications, or alternative treatments for menopause symptoms.

2. The Right to Privacy and Confidentiality

- Your medical information should be kept confidential under laws like the Health Insurance Portability and Accountability Act (HIPAA) in the United States.

- You are entitled to private consultations and control over who has access to your health records.

3. The Right to Access Medical Records

- You can request your medical history, test results, and treatment plans at any time.

- Reviewing your records can help you make informed decisions about your menopause management.

4. The Right to Participate in Treatment Decisions

- You have the right to ask questions, seek second opinions, and make decisions in line with your personal values and preferences.

- This is particularly important when exploring treatment options for menopausal symptoms, including both traditional and alternative therapies.

5. The Right to Respectful and Non-Discriminatory Care

- Healthcare providers must treat you with dignity, regardless of your age, gender, cultural background, or health status.

- You should not feel dismissed or minimized when discussing menopausal symptoms like hot flashes, sexual health, or emotional changes.

6. The Right to Refuse Treatment

- You are not obligated to undergo specific treatments and can decline tests, medications, or procedures if they do not align with your comfort level or beliefs.

7. The Right to Receive Clear Communication

- Your healthcare provider should explain diagnoses, treatment options, and procedures in clear, understandable terms.

- If something is unclear, you have to right to request more information or ask for explanations without feeling rushed or judged.

How to Advocate for Your Rights During Menopause Care

- Prepare for Appointments: Bring a list of questions and concerns to your medical appointments.

- Keep Records: Maintain a symptom journal and track treatments to provide your healthcare team with accurate information.

- Request Support: You can bring a trusted friend or family member to appointments if you feel more comfortable.

- Know Your Options: If a treatment recommendation does not feel right, you can seek a second opinion.

Understanding Insurance and Coverage

Next, let's talk about the labyrinthine world of insurance and coverage. It might not sound glamorous, but mastering this aspect ensures access to necessary care without undue financial strain. Who wants surprise bills or denied claims when you're juggling hot flashes and mood swings? A good guideline here is to dive into the nitty-gritty details of your insurance policy. Find out what your preventative care covers, which specialists are in your network, and what outpatient services you may need. With this knowledge, plan your appointments like a seasoned traveler, anticipating roadblocks and rerouting as needed.

Importantly, don't shy away from seeking help if you feel mistreated or discriminated against. Addressing discrimination fosters a better environment for you and paves the way for others who might walk the same path. Advocate for fair healthcare; plant seeds of change. For example, if a doctor dismisses your symptoms as "just menopause," challenge that narrative. Arm yourself with research, demand respect, and find allies among healthcare practitioners who genuinely listen.

Use the available support systems if you feel things are not right. Imagine trekking through a dense jungle—having a guide makes all the difference. Support groups, legal resources, and patient advocacy organizations act as your guides in the tangled web of healthcare disputes. If you ever face resistance or dismissal, reaching out to these networks will provide solace and actionable steps. They can offer insights on filing complaints and connect you with experts who can mediate conflicts and uphold your rights.

Building a strong support system extends beyond conflict resolution. It's about creating a community that uplifts and educates. Peer-led support groups, designed specifically for menopausal women, create spaces where women empower one another by sharing experiences, exchanging advice, and fostering collective wisdom. These communities reassure you that you're not isolated and validate your experiences while offering practical solutions.

Reflecting on these points, knowing your rights is integral to taking charge of your health. As a woman experiencing menopause, it's essential to transition from a passive recipient of care to an active participant. This proactive approach affects your well-being and influences systemic changes in healthcare delivery, ensuring future generations face fewer barriers.

Remember, you may ask questions, seek second opinions, and make informed choices about your body. Your voice matters, and exercising your rights plays a vital role in transforming healthcare interactions from transactional to relational. Whether it's negotiating with your insurance provider or addressing implicit biases in the consulting room, every step taken asserts your agency.

Creating a Personalized Wellness Plan

Menopause can feel like walking through a maze blindfolded. The secret to finding your way through this transition smoothly? Crafting a personalized wellness plan tailored to your needs, sprinkled with a hint of humor and patience. Let's break it down step by step.

First things first, self-reflection is your compass. Pondering your health priorities isn't just navel-gazing; it's your guide to crafting a wellness plan that's as unique as you are. What makes you tick? Is it yoga at sunrise or a cozy evening with a good book and herbal tea? List these priorities. Reflect on what brings you joy and balance, both physically and mentally. This introspection lays the groundwork for a purposeful wellness plan that resonates with your lifestyle and values.

Once you've got your list of priorities, it's time to enlist some expert advice. Collaboration with healthcare providers can refine your plan with valuable clinical insights. Think of them as your wellness sidekicks, ready to swoop in with research-backed guidance. Whether it's nutritional adjustments or tailored exercise routines, healthcare professionals can offer invaluable input to fine-tune your plan. It's like having a GPS for your health path—no more getting lost in the quagmire of internet advice.

Setting actionable steps involves breaking down your goals into bite-sized pieces. Small, realistic steps reduce being overwhelmed and keep you moving forward, like climbing a staircase one rung at a time rather than trying to leap straight to the top. If you want to exercise more, start with a brisk 10-minute walk and gradually extend it. Each tiny victory will fuel your motivation, making consistent progress achievable and rewarding.

As you start your wellness journey, remember that flexibility is imperative. Regular assessments are your check-ins, like pit stops on a long road trip, allowing you to review your route and make necessary adjustments. Maybe that yoga class isn't cutting it anymore, or you've discovered a new love for salsa dancing. Be open to change and willing to tweak your plan. This adaptability will ensure your wellness plan isn't static but develops as you do.

Finally, let's talk about celebrating victories and learning from setbacks. Every step forward, no matter how small, deserves acknowledgment. Did you manage to meditate three times this week? Give yourself a high five! If you stumble, don't be too hard on yourself—use it as a learning opportunity. Maybe that particular strategy didn't fit your lifestyle, or perhaps you're still adjusting. Welcome these moments and use them to strengthen your resolve.

Second Opinions: When "You're Fine" Doesn't Feel Right

"I'm sweating excessively at night, have memory loss, and experience extreme mood swings."

The doctor barely glances up from their clipboard. Smiling a smile that seems to come from a customer service manual, they say, "It's just stress. Or maybe your age. Have you tried yoga?"

You're not alone if you've ever wanted to flip a table and walk out mid-consultation. Many menopausal women have had their very real symptoms dismissed as normal aging or stress. And while deep breathing may be great for many things, it will not fix a raging hot flash or your vanishing libido.

So, when is enough *enough*?

The Moment You Know It's Time for a Second Opinion

Remember, you are the CEO of your health. Feeling unheard by your doctor? Get a second opinion.

Look out for these red flags:

- **Dismissive diagnoses:** If you're repeatedly told, "It's just stress" or "It's normal," with no investigation into your symptoms, it's a sign that your concerns aren't being taken seriously.

- **Quick fixes without explanations:** Suggesting lifestyle tweaks or medications without discussing the *why* behind your symptoms is a red flag.

- **Lack of menopause knowledge:** If your doctor seems uncomfortable or uninformed about menopause, it's not your job to educate them.

Options for a Second Opinion

So, you've decided to explore greener pastures. What next? Here are your options:

- **Menopause specialists:** Seek doctors who specialize in menopause or hormonal health. They'll likely know their way around an HRT conversation better than your current general practitioner.

- **Functional medicine practitioners:** For a more holistic approach, functional medicine practitioners focus on root causes and may explore both traditional and alternative options.

- **Women's health clinics:** Many larger cities and healthcare networks have clinics focused only on women's health, including menopause care.

- **Telehealth options: Virtual consultations with menopause specialists conveniently offer expert advice, especially when there are limited local options.**

- **Ask around:** Don't underestimate the power of the menopause grapevine. Friends, family, and even online forums can be great resources for finding a provider who "gets it."

Let's clarify: Seeking a second opinion doesn't mean betraying your current doctor. It means you value your health enough to keep looking until you find someone who values it, too. Here's how to do it guilt-free:

- **Frame it as a team effort:** You can politely say, "I'd like to explore this further and get another perspective."

- **Be direct:** "I feel like we haven't fully addressed my concerns, and I'd like to consult someone with more experience in menopause care."

- **Own it:** Your health, your rules. No explanations are required.

Before you walk into your next appointment, know what you want and write down your "non-negotiables" for care. This includes thorough investigation with tests to rule out other conditions and clear explanations of your options, respectful listening from a provider who won't interrupt or dismiss you, and a true partnership with someone willing to collaborate on a care plan that aligns with your goals and values.

If your new doctor ticks these boxes, congratulations—you've found a keeper! If not, remember: There's always another option, another opinion, and another opportunity to find someone who'll treat you like the powerhouse you are.

You've spent your whole life taking care of everyone else. It's your turn to be the priority. So speak up, buttercup. The right doctor is out there, and they'll be ready to listen, collaborate, and help you feel like yourself again—minus the midnight hot flash dance routines.

Bringing It All Together

This chapter has the essential strategies: building effective communication with healthcare providers, organizing your health records, and asking the right questions. You're actively engaging in your health journey with confidence and clarity   empowerment comes with reading glasses and a well-organized folder.

The secret to successful doctor visits? Preparation and candor. Approach appointments with your questions ready and don't be afraid to bring levity to the conversation. This openness transforms your healthcare provider from a distant authority into a trusted ally. As the protagonist of your health story, every conversation is a stepping stone toward solutions tailored to you. While menopause might throw a few curveballs your way, you're more than equipped to handle them.

Chapter Ten

Plot Twist: The Best Is Yet to Come

Menopause is like strolling through a theme park you never planned to visit. It's the one ride in life that never seems to follow the guidebook and has more twists than your favorite thriller novel. Enjoy the ride, gray streaks and all! After all, this whirlwind tour can be the gateway to a lifetime of embracing freedom, self-discovery, and undeniable strength. Menopause invites you to reshape your narrative, redefine beauty beyond skin-deep allure, and become your hero—no capes required!

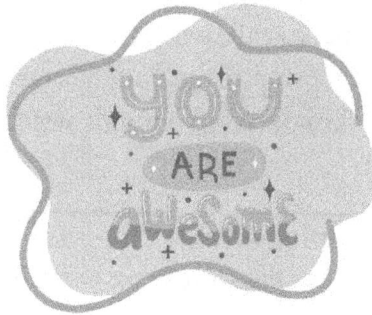

In this chapter, we'll explore how menopause, much like a pesky internet update, nudges us into introspection and personal growth, whether we're ready or not. Expect to venture into the world of redefining your identity when societal expectations no longer bind you and discover newfound passions that keep your spirit buoyant. From shaking off previous responsibilities to exploring hobbies that once gathered dust, you'll be reminded that reinvention isn't just possible; it's inevitable.

Reflecting on Personal Growth and Changes

Menopause is often viewed as a time filled with uncertainties and physical changes. However, it also presents an extraordinary opportunity for personal growth and self-discovery. Embracing the change can be empowering and transformative, leading to greater self-acceptance and understanding of one's evolution. This empowerment is a testament to your resilience and strength and a journey you're fully capable of handling.

Menopause encourages us to look inward and reflect on our identities. Like hitting the refresh button on life, this period allows you to reassess who you are and who you want to become. The process might begin with accepting the physical changes that accompany this transition. For instance, letting your hair turn gray naturally ("wisdom highlights," as I like to call them) can be a symbolic acceptance of aging with grace. It's a step toward self-acceptance, reminding us that beauty isn't just skin deep—it's about wisdom and experience, too.

Re-evaluating your identity during menopause can lead to the discovery of new passions. As life simplifies, with fewer responsibilities such as childcare, there's suddenly more time to explore interests previously pushed aside. Maybe it's picking up a paintbrush after years of driving a carpool. This time of life acts as a catalyst for rediscovering forgotten hobbies or trying new ones; such activities provide joy and a sense of fulfillment and purpose.

Appreciating how far you've traveled builds resilience. Life experiences are like chapters in a book, each with its lessons and stories, and reflecting on these experiences brings to light the strength and wisdom gained along the way. These reflections highlight how you overcame challenges in the past, reinforcing the belief that your current hurdles, including those encountered during menopause, can also be managed successfully. Every wrinkle or laughter line tells a story of triumph, hardship, laughter, and love—all vital components of who you are today.

Bring on the Growth Mindset

Viewing this phase as a chance to grow can help you manage the associated stresses and uncertainties. Instead of seeing menopause as an ending, consider it a beginning—a stage ripe with opportunities for self-exploration and understanding. Allowing yourself to sit with uncertainty opens the door to deeper insights about who you are and what matters most to you now.

One useful guideline for effectively accepting this transition is to build a growth mindset. This involves being open to learning from every experience, remaining flexible, and seeing challenges as opportunities rather than setbacks. It's about shifting perspectives from what may be lost to what can be gained. Engaging in mindfulness, meditation, or journaling practices can facilitate this mental shift, promoting peace and clarity amid change.

Consider incorporating mindfulness into your daily routines. Mindfulness can help ground you in the present, making it easier to reflect on emotions without judgment. It fosters a space to observe your thoughts and feelings, understand them better, and respond compassionately. Additionally, mindfulness has been shown to reduce stress, improve emotional regulation, and improve overall well-being—particularly valuable benefits during menopause.

As we've discussed, supporting one another during menopause can be incredibly rewarding. Sharing your experiences and insights with others going through similar changes creates a sense of community and belonging. Whether through support groups or casual meetups with friends, these interactions remind you that you're not alone and that many others are navigating this path together. This shared journey fosters a deep sense of understanding and support, making life's transitions smoother and more enjoyable.

Self-discovery involves courage and openness. It's about welcoming challenges and triumphs, accepting imperfections, and valuing progress over perfection. While challenging, menopause can be seen as an enriching experience when approached with curiosity and patience. It's a time to rewrite your story, celebrate the person you've become, and chart a course for the future with enthusiasm.

As you continue on this path, remember to practice patience and kindness toward yourself. Accept that it's okay not to have all the answers immediately. Life, much like menopause, is an ever-evolving process. The journey of continual self-discovery and growth enriches life, regardless of age or stage. Be kind to yourself, and remember that it's okay to take your time and enjoy the process.

Setting Goals for the Future

Establishing personal and health-related goals can be an empowering way to accept and welcome menopause as a positive transformation. Visioning the future is the first step; it's as if you're painting your masterpiece, with every brushstroke representing a goal toward a fulfilling life post-menopause. This visualization acts as a compass, providing the motivation and direction needed to navigate this period gracefully and purposefully.

Imagine clearly defining where you want to be in five, ten, or even fifteen years. This forward-thinking approach inspires and instills a sense of empowerment as you become the architect of your life's story. It's about looking beyond the changes and seeing the opportunities to shape a future that aligns with your aspirations and values.

Health and Lifestyle Goals

Regarding health and lifestyle goals, focusing on fitness is important to support long-term well-being during menopause. Engage in activities that keep you moving; make sure they include things you enjoy. Put an extra wiggle into folding the laundry, biking to the park, enjoying golf, or stretching out those muscles with wall Pilates. Finding what works best for you is so important. Not only do these exercises boost your physical health, but they also release happy hormones that uplift your mood. Setting realistic, achievable fitness goals, starting with small targets and building up over time, can maintain your motivation. Finally, tracking your progress can add a sense of accomplishment to these endeavors.

Nutrition, too, needs extra attention when you're managing your weight and overall health. Shoot for a balanced diet rich in whole grains, fruits, vegetables, and lean proteins. Adjust your caloric intake as your metabolism slows, being mindful of portion sizes. Staying hydrated is also essential, helping manage hunger and improve metabolism. These dietary strategies contribute to maintaining a healthy lifestyle post-menopause.

Pursuing Personal Aspirations

Pursuing personal aspirations is another key aspect of this phase. Have you considered learning a new skill, traveling to new places, or pursuing a long-held dream? Menopause provides the perfect opportunity to focus on your passions. Society often associates certain achievements or milestones with youth, but the truth is, there's no expiration date on ambition. This time of life is a chance to achieve dreams and ambitions like never before, driven by the wisdom and experience you've gained over the years. You're more equipped than ever to pursue what truly matters.

Building community connections and support systems can broaden your emotional resources and strengthen your networks during this transformative time. Friends, family, and community groups can provide vital support and encouragement, making menopause a little less of a hot mess (pun intended). Social connections build emotional well-being and reduce feelings of isolation. Engaging in shared activities, whether fitness classes, hobby clubs, or volunteer work, creates bonds that boost emotional resilience and enrich personal experiences.

Establishing social support networks is vital. Family members' participation, particularly partners' participation, in health promotion programs positively impacts women's quality of life post-menopause (Rostami-Moez et al., 2023). Their involvement can lead to greater improvements in both physical and mental health, ensuring a supportive and nurturing environment.

Celebrating Achievements and Resilience

Menopause is your personal hero's journey, where recognizing successes and celebrating milestones becomes essential in reinforcing a positive mindset and gratitude. Every step forward, no matter how small, is a victory worth acknowledging. Whether overcoming a hot flash in the middle of an important meeting or simply making it through the day with a smile, each success contributes to building resilience. Focusing on these achievements can create a sense of accomplishment that lifts your spirit and provides strength for future challenges.

Celebrating these moments doesn't have to be grandiose. Perhaps it's treating yourself to a spa day after surviving a particularly intense week, or maybe it's sharing a heartfelt dinner with friends who understand your triumphs and trials. It's about accepting the little joys, the "I did it!" moments that deserve to be honored. Remember to pat yourself on the back regularly. After all, if you don't celebrate your own wins, who will?

Sharing Resilience

Sharing stories of resilience among women has always been a powerful community-building tool. When women hear about others thriving despite the hurdles menopause presents, it inspires strength and offers validation. These stories create a blend of experiences, bringing together narratives of courage, fortitude, and perseverance. Sharing these tales could be as simple as organizing a meetup over coffee or an online forum where women share insights and experiences.

In these shared spaces, stories like Brenda's, who discovered new hobbies during menopause, or Mary's, who started her own business at 52, serve as hope. They remind everyone that menopause isn't the end, but the beginning of another exciting chapter. Through this communal storytelling, women build networks of support that corroborate their experiences and inspire each other to keep pushing forward.

Menopause Misdiagnosed: How Gina Became the Hero of Her Own Story

At 38, Gina's periods stopped, but life didn't pause. Raising her two-year-old daughter in rainy England, far from her Italian family, she was told by everyone—doctors, nurses, and family—that it was postpartum depression. Antidepressants became her daily routine, but Gina felt worse: foggy, moody, and crying in the grocery store over paper towels.

Two years of frustration later, Gina had a hunch: *Could this be menopause?* A quick Google search confirmed it was possible, and then a new doctor ordered tests and gave her the truth—peri-menopause, not depression. Gina cried, relieved to finally understand her body.

HRT brought clarity and balance. Gina felt like herself again, but she didn't stop there. She started a blog, *Hot Flashes and Cold Pasta*, humorously sharing her journey and building a community of women moving through the chaos of menopause. Her kitchen became the hub for "Menopause and Martinis" nights, filled with laughter and resilience.

By embracing the challenge, Gina turned her misdiagnosis into a mission, proving that menopause isn't just an ending—it's a powerful new chapter. As she told her mom, "We Italians thrive on drama—menopause is just another act."

Self-Compassion and Acceptance

Practicing self-compassion and acceptance during menopause is akin to watering a garden. The more kindness you extend toward yourself, the more emotional growth you build, allowing life's challenges to lead to profound self-discovery. This phase of life requires patience, gentleness, and an understanding that it's okay to have bad days and moments of doubt. Instead of criticizing yourself for imperfections, embracing your flaws and loving yourself despite them encourages healing and creates inner peace.

Imagine looking in the mirror each morning and extending words of kindness rather than criticism: "You're doing great," or "Today, I choose to be kind to myself." Such affirmations are tools of empowerment. Self-compassion turns struggles into stepping stones, transforming perceived weaknesses into strengths. By nurturing compassion within yourself, you open up pathways for emotional growth, ultimately guiding you toward a deeper understanding of who you are.

Creating celebratory rituals is perhaps one of the most joyful aspects of embracing menopause. These rituals don't require much effort but can improve your sense of achievement and strengthen your support networks. Whether lighting a candle to mark the start of a new month of menopausal adventures or throwing a themed party to honor the fact that you've overcome specific symptoms, these small acts serve big purposes. They offer opportunities to connect with others in meaningful ways, creating bonds that go beyond superficial interactions.

Incorporating these rituals into daily life brings about a sense of joy and camaraderie. Imagine inviting close friends over, sipping herbal tea under twinkling fairy lights while reminiscing about past adventures and future plans, or perhaps starting a journal where you jot down daily accomplishments and dreams—these practices allow you to reflect on your journey with pride and optimism.

Summary and Reflections

As you manage this midlife metamorphosis, think of it as the universe's quirky little gift—a time to hit pause and redefine yourself. Sure, there might be some hot flashes and unexpected joint pain, but it's also a chance to sow seeds for new adventures. This chapter has urged you to see menopause as an end to your reproductive years and an exciting kickoff to another vibrant stage. Welcome the changes like a new hobby; after all, who knows what hidden talents might emerge? It's about celebrating the wisdom you've gained—maybe with a few laughter lines or "wisdom highlights"—and owning this time in your life with all the grace and humor you've collected along the way.

Remember, you're part of a unique club where discussions about aging gracefully are encouraged and celebrated. This is a time to find joy in small victories and share stories of resilience, reinforcing that you're far from alone on this journey. So go on and add a splash of color to your life, whether it's through a new skill or deepening friendships. The world really is your oyster. By focusing on personal growth and learning to laugh at the quirks menopause throws your way, you'll continue to build a life narrative filled with strength, wisdom, and, undoubtedly, many more smiles.

Your Review Can Help Other Women

I hope you enjoyed *Menopause Doesn't Have to Suck.*

T hank you for reading my book! If my words have helped you on your menopause journey, would you consider taking a moment to share your thoughts? Your honest review helps other women find support during this important life transition and helps spread the message that **menopause doesn't have to suck!**

Please scan the QR code:

Join our Reader's Circle at www.sage-lifestyle-press.com for access to the advanced reader copies of upcoming books, free bonus downloads and guides, early access to special promotions, and helpful tips from our books to enhance your daily life. No spam, just inspiration, encouragement, and practical tools to help you thrive.

The Perimenopause Quick Guide

Are you wondering if what you're feeling is just stress or something else? Perimenopause is a stage that most women go through for 4 to 10 years before menopause, and its symptoms can be confusing if no one explains them. You might notice sleep issues, hot flashes, sudden anxiety, or brain fog that makes you doubt yourself. These changes are real; they have a biological cause, and you deserve clear information about what's happening in your body.

The Perimenopause Quick Guide is a free resource that explains everything in simple terms. Inside, you'll find a clear timeline to help you see where you are in the process, a list of common symptoms and their causes, and practical tips for sleep, nutrition, exercise, and mental health. There's also a symptom tracker to help you notice patterns and get ready to talk with your healthcare provider. Scan the QR code below to download your copy and start finding answers.

Conclusion

As you close this book, take a moment to reflect on what we've explored together. We've examined the intricacies of menopause while embracing it as an exciting chapter filled with possibility and humor. This isn't just about surviving—it's about thriving.

Picture menopause not as an ending but as a dawn of self-discovery. It's a reset button nudging you toward wisdom, strength, and potential that have always been there, waiting for their moment.

Knowledge has been our ally throughout these chapters. Understanding what's happening in your body gives you the tools to face each change with courage. You're no longer tiptoeing around menopause's mysteries—you're equipped with facts, ready to champion your health and advocate for yourself confidently.

Remember, you're not alone. There's comfort in knowing others have walked similar paths, many wearing the same humor-infused armor. Embrace the sisterhood of fellow menopause warriors eager to share insights, tears, and laughs. Revisit these sections whenever you need encouragement—this book remains your guide.

You've played a vital role by reading these pages. You're part of a movement rewriting the narrative, paving the way for future generations to approach menopause with joy and empowerment. If this book resonated with you, please share your experience through a review—your voice can light the path for someone else.

Here's to owning this adventure with strength and spunk. Here's to laughing at night sweats and wielding your beautiful self with grace and power. You've got this—not just menopause, but whatever life throws at you next. We're right here with you, rewriting menopause from a dreaded chapter into a tale of freedom and discovery. Cheers to you and all the glorious changes yet to unfold!

Appendix - The Science of Personalized Menopause Care

Your Genetic Blueprint: Why Menopause Hits Everyone Differently

E ver wonder why your sister sailed through menopause with barely a hot flash while you're melting through three shirts a day? Or why your friend's brain fog cleared up in six months, but yours has lingered for years? The answer might be written in your DNA.

We're entering an era where understanding your genetic makeup can help predict how menopause will affect you and what treatments are most likely to work. It's like having a preview instead of walking into the theater blind.

The Genetics of Hot Flashes

Some women experience hot flashes for a year or two. Others suffer for a decade or more. Researchers have identified genetic variants that influence hot flash severity and duration:

TACR3 Gene: Women with certain variants experience more frequent and severe hot flashes but tend to respond particularly well to treatments targeting the neurokinin 3 receptor (like fezolinetant). If you carry these variants, your doctor might skip straight to these medications instead of trying multiple other options first.

ESR1 Gene: This gene makes estrogen receptors. Different versions affect how sensitive your body is to estrogen—or the lack of it. Some variants are associated with more severe symptoms, while others seem protective. Women with certain variants might need higher or lower HRT doses to achieve relief.

Estrogen Metabolism Genes (CYP1A1 and CYP1B1): These control how your body processes estrogen. Some women break down estrogen quickly (fast metabolizers), while others process it slowly. This affects how long estrogen stays active in your system and can influence both symptom severity and treatment effectiveness.

What this means: In the near future, a genetic test might tell you, "You're likely to have severe hot flashes for 7-10 years, and you'll respond best to neurokinin antagonists or transdermal estrogen." No more trial and error.

Mood and Mental Health: Your Emotional Genetic Map

Depression and anxiety during menopause have strong genetic components:

Serotonin Transporter Gene (5-HTTLPR): Women with the short variant are significantly more likely to experience depression during menopause and tend to benefit from SSRIs for both mood symptoms and hot flashes. Knowing this ahead of time means you and your doctor can monitor mood symptoms closely and intervene early.

COMT Gene (The Warrior vs. Worrier Gene): This gene affects how your brain processes dopamine. Different variants are associated with either better stress tolerance or higher anxiety, helping predict whether you'll struggle more with anxiety or brain fog.

BDNF Gene: A common variant is associated with worse memory during menopause. Women with this variant might benefit more from cognitive training, exercise programs, and early HRT initiation.

Weight Gain: Why Your Sister Stays Slim

Several genes influence how menopause affects your metabolism:

FTO Gene: Certain variants make you more susceptible to weight gain during menopause, particularly belly fat. Women with high-risk variants might need more aggressive dietary interventions and exercise programs.

MC4R Gene: This regulates appetite and metabolism. Variants associated with increased hunger and slower metabolism can make menopausal weight management particularly challenging. If you carry these variants, you might benefit from appetite-regulating medications or specific dietary strategies.

Bone Health: Your Skeleton's Genetic Destiny

Osteoporosis risk has a strong genetic component:

VDR Gene (Vitamin D Receptor): This determines how well your body uses vitamin D to build bone. Some variants are associated with lower bone density and higher fracture risk. If you carry high-risk variants, you might need higher vitamin D doses or more aggressive bone-building treatments.

COL1A1 Gene: A specific variant increases fracture risk by up to 40%. Women with this variant might benefit from earlier bone density screening and more proactive treatment.

Using Genetics to Decide: Should You Take HRT?

Beyond determining which type of HRT and what dose, genetic testing can help answer a fundamental question: should you take HRT at all?

BRCA1/BRCA2: Women with these mutations have traditionally been told to avoid HRT. However, recent research suggests short-term, low-dose HRT may be safe for BRCA carriers, especially after risk-reducing surgeries. Genetic testing clarifies your specific risk profile.

Clotting Disorders: Genetic variants that increase blood clot risk (Factor V Leiden, prothrombin mutations) significantly affect HRT safety. Women with these variants have higher risk with oral estrogen, but transdermal estrogen (patches, gels) carries much lower clot risk.

Glossary

A MH (Anti-Müllerian Hormone): A hormone that indicates your ovarian reserve. Low levels suggest you're running low on eggs—your ovaries' way of sending a "going out of business" notice.

APOE4: A genetic variant that increases Alzheimer's risk and affects how your brain responds to estrogen during menopause. Like having a warning label that says "handle brain health with extra care."

Bioidentical hormones: Hormones that are molecularly identical to what your body produces naturally. The difference between a knock-off handbag and the real deal—but for your ovaries.

Biomarkers: Measurable indicators in your blood (like FSH, estradiol, AMH) that tell the story of your hormonal journey. Think of them as your body's text updates about what's happening inside.

Brain fog: That frustrating mental cloudiness where you forget words mid-sentence and wonder why you walked into a room. Often temporary, always annoying.

COMT gene: The "warrior vs. worrier" gene that affects how your brain handles stress and processes dopamine. Determines whether you're more anxious or more forgetful during menopause.

Critical window hypothesis: The theory that starting HRT early in menopause protects your brain, but starting too late might not help (or could even harm). Timing is everything—like watering a plant before it completely dies.

CYP450 genes: Genes that control how fast or slow your liver breaks down medications. Explains why your friend's antidepressant works great but yours makes you feel terrible.

DHEA (Dehydroepiandrosterone): A precursor hormone that your body converts into estrogen and testosterone. The Swiss Army knife of hormones—does a little bit of everything.

Estradiol (E2): The strongest and most common form of estrogen during your reproductive years. When this drops during menopause, it triggers most of menopause's greatest hits.

Fast metabolizers: People whose bodies break down medications so quickly that standard doses barely have time to work. Requires adjusted dosing for optimal results.

Fezolinetant (Veozah): A non-hormonal medication for hot flashes (FDA-approved 2023). Blocks the brain pathway that triggers hot flashes without using any hormones. Finally, a newcomer to the party.

FSH (Follicle-Stimulating Hormone): Your brain's increasingly desperate wake-up call to your ovaries. High levels (over 25-30 mIU/mL) mean your brain is yelling, but your ovaries aren't listening anymore.

Genitourinary syndrome of menopause (GSM): The medical term for vaginal and urinary changes during menopause—dryness, pain, frequent UTIs. Previously called "vaginal atrophy," but apparently that sounded too depressing.

Gut-brain axis: The communication superhighway between your digestive system and your brain. Explains why fixing your gut bacteria might improve your mood during menopause.

Hot flashes (vasomotor symptoms): Sudden waves of heat, sweating, and flushing caused by your hypothalamus misreading your body temperature. Can last from seconds to several minutes and occur multiple times daily.

HRT (Hormone Replacement Therapy): Treatment using estrogen (with or without progesterone) to relieve menopause symptoms. The most effective treatment for hot flashes, night sweats, and vaginal dryness.

Libido: Sexual desire and interest. Often decreases during menopause due to hormonal changes, but also influenced by sleep quality, stress, relationship dynamics, and overall health.

Microbiome: The 100 trillion bacteria living in your gut. They're like tiny roommates who affect your mood, metabolism, and menopause symptoms—for better or worse.

MTHFR gene: A gene that affects how your body processes folate (vitamin B9), which is crucial for making mood-regulating neurotransmitters. About 40% of people have variants that reduce enzyme function.

Neurokinin 3 receptor: The brain receptor that triggers hot flashes. The newest medications block this receptor, turning off the hot flash signal without affecting hormones.

Neuroprotection: Strategies to protect your brain from age-related cognitive decline. During menopause, this might include HRT timing, exercise, diet, and sleep optimization.

Night sweats: Hot flashes that occur during sleep, often severe enough to drench your pajamas and sheets. The nocturnal version of hot flashes that ruins a good night's rest.

Osteoporosis: A condition where bones become weak and brittle due to decreased bone density. Risk increases significantly after menopause when estrogen levels drop.

Perimenopause: The transitional phase before menopause when your ovaries gradually produce less estrogen. Can last 4-10 years and often brings irregular periods and unpredictable symptoms.

Pharmacogenetic testing: Genetic testing that predicts how you'll respond to medications before you take them. Eliminates the medication roulette game.

Poor metabolizers: People whose bodies break down medications very slowly, causing drugs to build up to potentially toxic levels. Requires lower medication doses.

Prebiotics: Non-digestible fibers that feed your beneficial gut bacteria. Like fertilizer for the good bacteria in your microbiome.

Precision psychiatry: Using genetic testing to match people with the psychiatric medications most likely to work for them. No more trying five antidepressants before finding one that helps.

Progesterone: A hormone that prepares the uterus for pregnancy and regulates the menstrual cycle. In HRT, it protects the uterine lining from overgrowth caused by estrogen.

Psychobiotics: Probiotics specifically shown to improve mood, anxiety, or stress. Your gut bacteria as tiny therapists.

PT-141 (Bremelanotide): An FDA-approved injection for low sexual desire in women. Works on your brain's melanocortin receptors, not your hormones. Self-injected 45 minutes before anticipated intimacy.

Sarcopenia: Age-related muscle loss that typically begins around age 30 and accelerates after 60. Regular strength training helps combat it.

SERMs (Selective Estrogen Receptor Modulators): Medications that act like estrogen in some body parts (like bones) while blocking estrogen in others (like breast tissue). The smart bouncers of hormone therapy.

Serotonin transporter gene (5-HTTLPR): A gene that affects your risk of depression during menopause and how well you'll respond to antidepressants. Comes in "short" and "long" variants.

SHBG (Sex Hormone Binding Globulin): A protein that binds up sex hormones (especially testosterone) and makes them unavailable for use. High levels mean your hormones are locked up and can't work.

TACR3 gene: A gene that affects hot flash severity. Certain variants mean you're in for more intense vasomotor symptoms.

Testosterone: Often called the "male hormone," but women produce it too (just in smaller amounts). Affects energy, muscle mass, bone density, and libido. Levels decline with age and menopause.

TSEC (Tissue-Selective Estrogen Complex): A combination of estrogen plus a SERM that provides multiple benefits with fewer risks. Like getting the advantages of HRT without needing a separate pill to protect your uterus.

Vaginal atrophy: See Genitourinary syndrome of menopause (GSM).

Vaginal laser therapy: Fractional CO2 laser treatment that stimulates collagen production and tissue regeneration in vaginal tissue. A non-hormonal option for treating GSM symptoms.

VDR gene (Vitamin D Receptor): Determines how well your body uses vitamin D to build bone. Some variants increase osteoporosis risk after menopause and may require higher vitamin D supplementation.

References

Albert, K. M., & Newhouse, P. A. (2019). Estrogen, stress, and depression: Cognitive and biological interactions. *Annual Review of Clinical Psychology, 15*, 399–423. https://doi.org/10.1146/annurev-clinpsy-050718-095557

American College of Obstetricians and Gynecologists. (n.d.). *Hormone therapy for menopause.* Retrieved March 2, 2025, from https://www.acog.org/womens-health/faqs/hormone-therapy-for-menopause

American Heart Association. (n.d.). *Menopause and cardiovascular risk.* Go Red for Women. Retrieved March 3, 2025, from https://www.goredforwomen.org/en/know-your-risk/menopause/menopause-and-cardiovascular-risk

Aninye, I. O., Laitner, M. H., & Shivani, C. (2021). Menopause preparedness: Perspectives for patient, provider, and policymaker consideration. *Journal of the Menopause Society, 28*(10), 1186–1191. https://doi.org/10.1097/gme.0000000000001819

Ardeljan, A. D., & Hurezeanu, R. (2023). *Sarcopenia.* StatPearls Publishing. https://www.ncbi.nlm.nih.gov/books/NBK560813/

Avis, N. E., Crawford, S. L., & Greendale, G. (2021). Study of Women's Health Across the Nation (SWAN): Overview of the cohort, research findings, and future directions. *Menopause, 28*(8), 937–951.

Bansal, R., & Aggarwal, N. (2019). Menopausal hot flashes: A concise review. *Journal of Mid-Life Health, 10*(1), 6–13. https://doi.or g/10.4103/jmh.JMH_7_19

Berin, E., Hammar, M., Lindblom, H., Lindh-Åstrand, L., Rubér, M., & Spetz Holm, A.-C. (2019). Resistance training for hot flushes in postmenopausal women: A randomized controlled trial. *Maturitas, 126*, 55–60. https://doi.org/10.1016/j.maturitas.2019.05.005

Biglia, N., Bounous, V. E., De Seta, F., Lello, S., Nappi, R. E., & Paoletti, A. M. (2019). Non-hormonal strategies for managing menopausal symptoms in cancer survivors: An update. *ecancer, 13*, 909. https://ecancer.org/en/journal/article/909

Bousman, C. A., et al. (2021). Review and consensus on pharmacogenomic testing in psychiatry. *Pharmacopsychiatry, 54*(1), 5–17. https://doi.org/10.1055/a-1254-2225

British Heart Foundation. (n.d.). *Menopause and heart disease.* Retrieved March 2, 2025, from https://www.bhf.org.uk/informationsupport/support/wom en-with-a-heart-condition/menopause-and-heart-disease

Brodhead, H. (2021, June 23). *Estrogen, progesterone, testosterone: Side effects & safety.* Healing Roots Medicine. https://www.healingrootsmedicine.com/post/estrogen-proge sterone-testosterone-side-effects-safety

Catalyst. (n.d.). *Stop the stigma: Addressing menopause in the workplace.* https://www.catalyst.org/research/address-menopause-stigm a/

Centers for Disease Control and Prevention. (2024). *Women and heart disease.* https://www.cdc.gov/heart-disease/about/women-an d-heart-disease.html

Choe, S.-A., & Sung, J. (2020). Trends of premature and early menopause: A comparative study of the U.S. and Korea National Health and Nutrition Examination Surveys. *Journal of Korean Medical Science, 35*(16), e97. https://doi.org/10.3346/jkms.2020.35.e97

Cleveland Clinic. (n.d.). *Hormone therapy for menopause symptoms.* https://my.clevelandclinic.org/health/treatments/15245-hor mone-therapy-for-menopause-symptoms

Cohen, S. (2023, October 24). *Treating the mental health side of menopause.* UCLA Health. https://www.uclahealth.org/news/arti cle/treating-mental-health-side-menopause

Dąbrowska-Galas, M., Dąbrowska, J., Ptaszkowski, K., & Plinta, R. (2019). High physical activity level may reduce menopausal symptoms. *Medicina, 55*(8), 466. https://doi.org/10.3390/medicina550 80466

Drake, C. L., et al. (2019). Treating chronic insomnia in post-menopausal women: A randomized clinical trial comparing CBT-I, sleep restriction therapy, and sleep hygiene education. *Sleep, 42*(2), zsy217. https://doi.org/10.1093/sleep/zsy217

Erdélyi, A., et al. (2024). The importance of nutrition in menopause and perimenopause—A review. *Nutrients, 16*(1), 27. https://doi.or g/10.3390/nu16010027

Ghada AlSwayied, Frost, R., & Hamilton, F. L. (2024). Menopause knowledge, attitudes, and experiences of women in Saudi Arabia: A qualitative study. *BMC Women's Health, 24*, 624. https://doi.org/ 10.1186/s12905-024-03456-7

Goins, S. (2023, October 18). *Mayo Clinic minute: Managing sleep during menopause.* Mayo Clinic News Network. https://newsnetwork.mayoclinic.org/discussion/mayo-clinic-minute-managing-sleep-during-menopause/

Goldstein, J. M. (2021, November 3). *Menopause and memory: Know the facts.* Harvard Health Publishing. https://www.health.harvard.edu/blog/menopause-and-memory-know-the-facts-202111032630

Haufe, A., & Leeners, B. (2023). Sleep disturbances across a woman's lifespan: The role of reproductive hormones. *Journal of the Endocrine Society, 7*(5), bvad036. https://doi.org/10.1210/jendso/bvad036

Holland, K. (2024, July 17). *Osteoporosis, bone health, and menopause.* Healthline. https://www.healthline.com/health/menopause/osteoporosis

Johns Hopkins Medicine. (n.d.). *Menopause and the cardiovascular system.* Retrieved March 2, 2025, from https://www.hopkinsmedicine.org/health/conditions-and-diseases/menopause-and-the-cardiovascular-system

Kostis, J. B., & Wilson, A. C. (2020). Changes in cardiovascular risk factors during the menopause transition: The Framingham Heart Study. *Journal of the American Heart Association, 9*(20), e016494. https://doi.org/10.1161/JAHA.120.016494

Marcin, A. (2024, October 21). *What causes menopause brain fog, and how is it treated?* Healthline. https://www.healthline.com/health/menopause/menopause-brain-fog

Menopause Foundation of Canada. (2024, October 2). *Destigmatizing menopause becomes business critical as employers lose half a million days of productivity.* https://menopausefoundationcanada.ca/worl d-menopause-month-2024

Miller, S. (2024, January 11). *The truth about menopause: Debunking six common misconceptions.* Jefferson Health. https://www.jeffersonhealth.org/your-health/living-well/t he-truth-about-menopause-misconceptions

National Cancer Institute. (n.d.). *Menopausal hormone therapy and cancer risk.* U.S. Department of Health and Human Services. Re-trieved March 3, 2025, from https://www.cancer.gov/about-cancer /causes-prevention/risk/hormones/mht-fact-sheet

National Institute on Aging. (n.d.). *What is menopause?* https://w ww.nia.nih.gov/health/menopause/what-menopause

NHS Inform. (2024, July 23). *Menopause.* https://www.nhsinform.scot/healthy-living/womens-health/later-y ears-around-50-years-and-over/menopause-and-post-menopause-he alth/menopause/

Office on Women's Health. (2023, January 6). *Menopause and sex-uality.* U.S. Department of Health and Human Services. https://w ww.womenshealth.gov/menopause/menopause-and-sexuality

Peacock, K., Carlson, K., & Ketvertis, K. (2023). *Menopause.* Stat-Pearls Publishing. https://www.ncbi.nlm.nih.gov/books/NBK507 826/

Williamson, L. (2023, February 20). *The connection between menopause and cardiovascular disease risks.* American Heart Associ-ation. https://www.heart.org/en/news/2023/02/20/the-connectio n-between-menopause-and-cardiovascular-disease-risks

Youngblood Gregory, S. (2024, March 28). *The health benefits of humor.* Mayo Clinic Press. https://mcpress.mayoclinic.org